Essentials of Gestalt Theoretical Psychotherapy

Essentials of Gestalt Theoretical Psychotherapy

Edited by Gerhard Stemberger

Co-authored by
Doris Beneder, Angelika Böhm, Thomas Fuchs,
Bernadette Lindorfer, Edward S. Ragsdale, Gerhard Stemberger,
Katharina Sternek, Elena & Giancarlo Trombini, Andrzej Zuczkowski

Published by the
Austrian Association for Gestalt Theoretical Psychotherapy
Österreichische Arbeitsgemeinschaft für Gestalttheoretische Psychotherapie

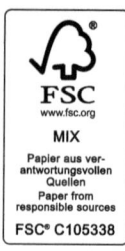

Impressum

Bibliografische Information der Deutschen Nationalbibliothek: Die Deutsche Nationalbibliothek verzeichnet diese Publikation in der Deutschen National-bibliografie; detaillierte bibliografische Daten sind im Internet über dnb.dnb.de abrufbar.

© 2022 Gerhard Stemberger als Herausgeber und die Autorinnen und Autoren der Einzel-Beiträge

Printed and published by: BoD - Books on Demand, Norderstedt

ISBN: 9783756209064

CONTENTS

Overview and Introduction (*Gerhard Stemberger*) ..... p. 7

1. Psychotherapy: The Challenge and Power of Consistency
   (*Gerhard Stemberger*) ..... p. 13

2. Critical Realism: The Epistemic Position of Gestalt Theoretical
   Psychotherapy (*Katharina Sternek*) ..... p. 21

3. Personality Theory in Gestalt Theoretical Psychotherapy: Kurt Lewin's
   Field Theory and his Theory of Systems in Tension Revisited
   (*Bernadette Lindorfer*) ..... p. 34

4. Ego and Self in Gestalt Theory (*Gerhard Stemberger*) ..... p. 51

5. Basic Principles for Therapeutic Relationship and Practice in
   Gestalt Theoretical Psychotherapy (*Angelika Böhm*) ..... p. 70

6. "The way you make me feel" – Feeling-causality in language
   communication (*Andrzej Zuczkowski and Gerhard Stemberger*) ..... p. 86

7. The Task of Diagnostics in Gestalt Theoretical Psychotherapy
   (*Doris Beneder and Bernadette Lindorfer*) ..... p. 108

8. Gestalt Theoretical Psychotherapy – A Clinical Example
   (*Thomas Fuchs*) ..... p. 115

9. Reconciliation of Time Perspectives as a Criterion for Therapy Completion
   (*Giancarlo Trombini, Elena Trombini and Gerhard Stemberger*) ..... p. 126

10. Relational Determination in Interpersonal and Intrapsychic Experience
    (*Edward S. Ragsdale*) ..... p. 142

Bibliography ..... p. 165

About the Authors ..... p. 181

Overview and Introduction

Gerhard Stemberger

This is not a "How to..." book. Its focus is not on any particular therapeutic techniques or special new suggestions, which mental illnesses could be hidden here and there, and how to deal with them. Instead, it introduces basic ideas and concepts that theoretically "underlie" a particular understanding and method of psychotherapy - that is, ideas that are "behind" how Gestalt-theoretical psychotherapists see themselves and their clients, their problems in life, and how to face these problems together. This thorough reflection on what ideas of man and his life are behind this method of therapy is perhaps somewhat unusual, and for some readers, perhaps challenging. But we think it is necessary to come to more than a quick but superficial understanding, and it is worth the effort.

The reader for whom English is the native tongue may forgive the weaknesses of the language in this book. With one exception (Ed Ragsdale), English is a foreign language for all the other authors of this book, and they themselves suffer from the fact that here they lack the more sophisticated and beautiful expressive possibilities of their mother tongue. Nevertheless, they have tried to make their ideas understandable to people who are not native speakers of German or Italian, and they hope for the patience and linguistic sensitivity of their readers.

The current volume builds on the first-time introduction of basic concepts of GTP in English, as presented at the 21st Scientific Conference of the GTA "Motion – Spaces of Human Experience," 13th–15th June 2019, Warsaw, Poland, and subsequently published by *Sciendo* (a De Gruyter company) in a thematic issue of the Open Access e-journal *Gestalt Theory* (vol. 43, issue 1/2021: https://sciendo.com/issue/GTH/43/1). To promote and facilitate communication and exchange with colleagues from the psychotherapeutic field who do not speak German, ÖAGP has decided to present this collection - somewhat revised and expanded by additional contributions - now in the form of this printed workbook.[1]

---

[1] We thank Ed Ragsdale and Ian Verstegen for their help in reviewing some of the manuscripts and their suggestions for possible language improvements. They are in no way responsible for the remaining deficiencies.

The current volume presents some essential basic concepts of Gestalt Theoretical Psychotherapy in a coherent compilation[2]. A side effect of such a systematic presentation might be that it also helps to avoid the frequent confusion with Gestalt therapy, which has a similar sounding name, but in most of its forms – there are exceptions – differs substantially in its basic concepts. (A brief note on the history of Gestalt Theoretical Psychotherapy is given in the annex to this introduction.)

Ten contributions by authors from Austria, Italy, Germany, and the United States:

1. The papers on various core concepts of GTP and related subjects are preceded by a rationale and discussion of the importance of **consistency** in the substantive orientation of a psychotherapy method: "The power and challenge of consistency", by Gerhard Stemberger. Such consistency is not a mere theoretical-scientific matter, but a requirement of the nature of man and his life.

2. Because of the elementary role of cognitive processes for human experience and behavior, the second paper in the current volume highlights the **epistemological orientation** of Gestalt Theoretical Psychotherapy, which underlies all sub-concepts of the method from personality theory to praxeology: "Critical Realism: The Epistemic Position of Gestalt Theoretical Psychotherapy", by Katharina Sternek.

3. Psychotherapy is an intentional, planned, interactional process that implies that the therapist has assumptions about the human person and its functioning and about the nature and functioning of such an interactional process. Bernadette Lindorfer's third contribution in this volume deals with a core piece of **personality theory** in Gestalt Theoretical Psychotherapy: "Personality Theory in Gestalt Theoretical Psychotherapy: Kurt Lewin's Field Theory and his Theory of Systems in Tension Revisited".

4. Lindorfer's contribution on personality theory is complemented by a critical synopsis and further development of the views on **ego and self** in Gestalt psychology and their heuristic potential for psychotherapy: "Ego and Self in Gestalt theory" (G. Stemberger).

---

[2] Up to now, there have only been scattered publications on individual aspects of the field of Gestalt Theoretical Psychotherapy in English: H.-J. P. Walter's contributions on the compatibility of Gestalt theory and cognitive behavioral therapy (1997) and of Gestalt theory and Gestalt therapy (1999; cf. on this topic also Wollants 2008/2012 and Ragsdale 2010); M. Ruh (1999) and G. Stemberger (2008) on the issue of diagnostics in Gestalt Theoretical Psychotherapy; K. Sternek (2007) on the relationship of Gestalt psychology and attachment theory; U. Wedam (2007) and S. Wieltschnig (2016) on trauma therapy.

8

5. The frame of reference in which the practical procedures in psychotherapy acquire their meaning and develop their effectiveness is the relationship between therapist and client in the particular therapeutic situation. This is the focus of Angelika Böhm's contribution which outlines the understanding of the **therapeutic relationship and praxeology** in Gestalt Theoretical Psychotherapy and explains the main features of its therapeutic practice: "Basic Principles for Therapeutic Relationship and Practice in Gestalt Theoretical Psychotherapy".

6. "The way you make me feel" – **Feeling-causality in language communication** by Andrzej Zuczkowski and Gerhard Stemberger sheds light on the role of phenomenal causality of feelings, as experienced by people and expressed linguistically. In many situations, it determines their experience and behavior in interpersonal relationships. Thus, the great importance of language in life and psychotherapy is demonstrated by the example of emotional life.

7. Doris Beneder and Bernadette Lindorfer present the basic ideas of **diagnostics** in Gestalt Theoretical Psychotherapy as a process that primarily aims to enable the client to become a constructive diagnostician of her situation, the possibilities it offers, and the resources available for coping with it.

8. Taking the example of specific Gestalt theoretical approaches to **understand anorexia using the multiple-field approach**, Thomas Fuchs explains some aspects of Gestalt theoretical psychotherapeutic practice: "Gestalt Theoretical Psychotherapy - A Clinical Example".

9. Psychoanalyst and Gestalt psychologist Giancarlo Trombini (in collaboration with Elena Trombini and Gerhard Stemberger) presents possibilities of a Gestalt theoretical **analysis of the progression of psychotherapies**, offering central criteria for the decision on the completion of therapies based on Gestalt psychological concepts: "Reconciliation of Time Perspectives as a Criterion for Therapy Completion".

10. Edward Ragsdale concludes the thematic focus of the current volume with an exposition and discussion of one of the most fundamental principles of any Gestalt-theory based psychotherapy: "**Relational Determination** in Interpersonal and Intrapsychic Experience."

The reader may feel invited to send the editor and the authors her/his critical objections and own ideas on the topics touched upon in the contributions to this volume:

c/o Dr. Gerhard Stemberger

Email: gst@gestalttheory.net

Annex:
A brief note on the history of Gestalt Theoretical Psychotherapy

The history of the clinical-psychotherapeutic application of Gestalt theory cannot be adequately presented within the narrow confines of this introduction. I must limit myself to some necessarily highly abbreviated remarks.[3]

In the now more than 100-year history of Gestalt theory, this approach has radiated from its beginnings to a multitude of people working in clinical psychotherapy and the "schools of therapy" developed or represented by them. It did so in interaction with similarly directed scientific developments and new orientations of its time, which above all had in common the aim of overcoming mechanistic conceptions of life and man and the search for more appropriate holistic-dynamic alternatives (cf. Ash 1995, Harrington 1996, King & Wertheimer 2005). For example, people trained and inspired by Gestalt theory significantly influenced the development of group psychoanalysis, psychoanalytic psychotherapy, hypnotherapy, and catathym imaginative psychotherapy, various methods associated with humanistic psychology from Rogers' client-centered approach to Gestalt therapy and Moreno's psychodrama, to name a few. In this broader sense, then, psychotherapy based on or inspired by Gestalt theory has been around for more than 100 years. However, this early history of Gestalt theory in psychotherapy consisted, on the one hand, in the insertion of certain ideas and concepts, procedures, and research findings from Gestalt theory into other ideas, whereby these adoptions were often not insignificantly distant from their origin; on the other hand, in the personal integration of Gestalt theoretical thought into therapeutic practice by individual clinically active Gestalt psychologists who never set themselves the task of systematically formulating the basic concepts of their Gestalt theory based psychotherapeutic work. (e.g. Levy, Luchins, Harrower).

The impetus for such a formulation and thus for a Gestalt Theoretical Psychotherapy in the narrower sense was given a little more than 40 years ago by a small group of psychotherapists in Germany around Hans-Jürgen P. Walter and Rainer Kästl within the framework of the GTA, which they co-founded in 1979. Walter had previously presented a first outline of a Gestalt theoretical rationale for the integrative application of Gestalt therapy, psychodrama, talk therapy, depth psychology, behavior therapy, and group dynamics in 1977. Since then, the focus of further development and application of Gestalt Theoretical Psychotherapy has increasingly shifted to Austria, the motherland of so

---

[3] For a more detailed account, we refer to the chapter "Anwendungen der Gestalttheorie in der Psychotherapie," in Kästl & Stemberger 2011, 27-47, and for an account of the development of Gestalt Theoretical Psychotherapy within the GTA to Stemberger 2019.

many psychotherapy methods in history. It is now being further developed there by the Austrian Association for Gestalt Theoretical Psychotherapy (ÖAGP) with the GTA as its scientific umbrella organization, integrating the impulses of other Gestalt-psychologically oriented clinicians from other countries - among them especially from Italy (e.g., Giuseppe Galli, Anna Arfelli Galli, Giancarlo Trombini, Andrzej Zuczkowski).

1. Psychotherapy: The challenge and power of consistency

Gerhard Stemberger[4]

Summary:

As an introduction to the current volume, this article substantiates the possibility and meaningfulness of a coherent theoretical system for psychotherapy, as it is strived for in Gestalt Theoretical Psychotherapy and presented in several articles in this issue. The necessity of consistency in the theoretical assumptions and concepts of a psychotherapy method is not derived from scientific considerations alone, but already arises from the elementary role of consistency in human life. This also results in requirements for the consistency of theoretical foundations of psychotherapy. It is not fulfilled in a mere internal, logical consistency of its models, but only in the actual fitting together with the critical-phenomenal and naïve-phenomenal worlds of the therapists and their clients (in interaction with their „ naïve psychologies") in the reality test of life.

Such a coherent presentation of basic theoretical concepts as it is aimed for in the current volume has an implication that will be made explicit in the following introduction to this thematic focus: Namely, that consistency in thought and behavior plays a key role in human life – and therefore also a theoretical conception of psychotherapy needs consistency.

Psychotherapy rooted in the overall system of Gestalt theory

Gestalt Theoretical Psychotherapy (GTP) sees itself as a method of psychotherapy that bases its theoretical assumptions not only on *partial* theses and *partial* findings *of* Gestalt psychology, as we find in various other schools of psychotherapy, but tries to apply in a consistent way the *overall system* of Gestalt theory of the Berlin School (Wertheimer, Köhler, Koffka, Lewin and others).

That this is possible at all presupposes that Gestalt psychology (or more precisely: the Gestalt theory of the Berlin School) *is* actually an organized system whose various sub-approaches are systematically related to each other.

According to Wolfgang Metzger and Paul Tholey one can name five such subsystems of Gestalt theory: Gestalt psychology as *methodology* (holistic view and experimental orientation), Gestalt psychology as *phenomenology* (a wealth of research-backed knowledge about Gestalt phenomena in perception and cognition, behavior and life processes, including social relations), Gestalt psychology as a *theory of dynamic processes* (from productive thought to the psychology of will and social life), Gestalt psychology as a *psychophysical approach* (including the working hypothesis of isomorphism), and - permeating the four

---

[4] Revised version of the editorial for the special issue "Essentials of Gestalt Theoretical Psychotherapy" of the journal *Gestalt Theory*, 43(1), 1-12.

sub-approaches mentioned above - Gestalt psychology as an *epistemological approach* (critical realism).

These five subsystems of Gestalt theory are mutually dependent and support each other (cf. Stemberger 2020a). Whoever takes only partial aspects from this overall system accepts substantial losses. For example, Gestalt theory shares a holistic orientation with numerous other systems; detached from the experimental orientation of Gestalt psychology, however, the holistic attitude loses the possibility to determine the reach and limits of what the whole in the concrete case *is* and what holds it together as a whole. A speculative "everything is somehow connected with everything" then easily takes the place of a clarification of the concrete connections in the specific case.

On consistency in psychotherapy concepts

Nevertheless, it would have little relevance to strive for consistency in the formulation of the theoretical foundations of one's psychotherapy method if consistency did not also have corresponding significance in the actual life of human beings. This conviction is among the most fundamental in Gestalt theory. According to this view, the striving for consistency is part of and an expression of the basic dynamic ordering principle that has been identified in Gestalt theory as the striving for Prägnanz, the umbrella term for the so-called „Gestalt laws" or – as Max Wertheimer called them in his groundbreaking work of 1923 – the *Gestalt factors*. Metzger formulates on this principle pointedly: "The urge to fix what is in disorder and to be an obstetrician to what is undeveloped is undoubtedly one of man's deepest drives......." (Metzger 2001, 232; transl. GSt; for a discussion of the Prägnanz principle see Luccio 2019)

In many schools of psychotherapy, echoing this and kindred thoughts, one finds similar emphases on the role of consistency in the life of man. One thinks, for example, of the pursuit of meaning in Adler's (individual psychology) and Frankl's (logotherapy and existential analysis) therapy systems. Or the idea of the necessary integration of the personality during individuation in C.G. Jung's therapy system, where personality integration and maturation is reached by overcoming inconsistencies between the individual and collective unconscious. One thinks, to add a further example, of C. Rogers' call for overcoming the incongruity hampering the unfolding of the personality, the necessity to close the gap between the „real self" and the „ideal self", between the "I am" and the "I should"; and one thinks of his „Necessary and Sufficient Conditions of Therapeutic Personality Change", with the dual emphasis on the importance of congruence, both on the side of the client and on the side of the therapist. Common to all these approaches, albeit in different forms, is the conviction that consistency is essential to human life and that supporting the pursuit of it is one of the core tasks of psychotherapy.

A key question in this context, however, is: What does the respective consistency claim refer to? *What is* something supposed to be consistent with?

Probably the most elementary claim to consistency for human life is that of the matching of our individual phenomenal world of experience with the extra-phenomenal reality which we share with other human beings. Human life and coexistence in society and shared natural environment would not be possible if veridicality of our perceptual world would not be given to a very high degree. Even more: The dynamic peculiarities of our phenomenal world described by Gestalt theory make this phenomenal microcosm even "super-veridical" - it is not only able to represent the realities of the extra-phenomenal world to a large extent accurately, it can furthermore grasp their meaning, function and valence for the respective human being; this is more essential for the life of the human being and thus more veridical than the completely exact representation of the other physical features of the extra-phenomenal world.

Inconsistency in life

Even in the simplest everyday experience, however, one repeatedly encounters inconsistencies, facts that do not fit together for oneself in the given situation. One may feel compelled to review one's perception and one's previous models of understanding and explaining the given facts and relationships. Especially if this concerns one's most important interpersonal relationships, the task of gaining a new consistency of one's world and oneself within this world may put oneself to a hard test. Already the earliest Gestalt theoretical works on psychopathology, still initiated by Max Wertheimer himself, illuminated these connections between the demand for consistency and mental health in their essential outlines (see Schulte 1924; Levy 1943; Levy 1986). Failure to meet the requirement of consistently in reordering one's life and one's view of it, especially after crises, can lead to great psychological distress (and thus to psychotherapy). During or in the wake of such a crisis "detailed processes must take place again and again if the recentering is to result in a liveable, concrete, and consistent view of life and world, compatible with the objective data and structures of the world, as well as with the psychological needs of the person. " (Levy 1943, 66f)

However, we know that people often differ quite widely in whether they perceive something as inconsistent at all. And also, the reaction of humans to the finding of inconsistencies in their world can turn out quite differently. Leon Festinger, for example, has put forward the thesis (still popular today) that humans, when confronted with inconsistencies in their world, tend to eliminate the resulting "cognitive dissonance" by restructuring and reinterpretation (Festinger 1957). In my opinion, Solomon Asch was right when he rejected this notion (Asch 1959). That the modes of reaction described by Festinger exist and that this can also lead the striving for consistency astray, all this is undisputed. However, if this were the dominating basic tendency of man, there would have been no further development of mankind at all - only the perception of inconsistencies and the confrontation with them enables further development, be it in science, be it in the individual life of man. Man's striving for consistency is both a challenge and a powerful driving force, in coping with everyday life as well as in psychotherapy.

If one looks at the theory systems of the various psychotherapeutic schools, it is not unusual for their development that from time to time they contain concepts and approaches that are incompatible with each other. Giuseppe Galli points to a historical example of this in the development of psychoanalysis: "While Freud based therapeutic treatment on the relational and dialogical method, the theory was created with building blocks that were characterized by a monopersonal way of thinking. However, this contradiction between theory and practice in Freud was overcome by some of his followers through the application of a relational model." (Galli 1997 in 2017, 109)

In the development of Gestalt theory, too, such inconsistencies have repeatedly come to light. Wolfgang Köhler, for example, has pointed out that even core theses of Gestalt theory, such as the understanding of the striving for Prägnanz, had to be corrected over time compared to their beginnings, because their original understanding could not explain certain phenomena without contradictions (Köhler 1951/1993). Giuseppe Galli, on the other hand, has pointed out other inconsistencies in the course of the development of Gestalt theory - where its relational approach was not consistently implemented, for example in the sometimes one-sided attention to the object side of the field of experience, or where, for example, Lewin's model of life space, by neglecting the psychophysical connections, did not fit together with his discoveries on interpersonal processes and group dynamics (see on this Galli 1997 and Lindorfer in the present issue of this journal).

"Naïve psychology" and therapeutic concepts

The contributions in this volume show the effort to achieve the greatest possible consistency of the presented basic concepts of Gestalt Theoretical Psychotherapy (GTP), on the one hand, regarding their internal conceptual consistency, and on the other hand, regarding the correspondence with today's realities of life of psychotherapists and clients in our time and our world.

Especially the work of the Gestalt psychologist Fritz Heider (Heider 1958[5]) reminds us, however, of another, ultimately even decisive dimension of the requirement of consistency. Insofar as the explanatory and orientational models of psychotherapy theory find their way at all into the everyday consciousness of the therapists and their clients (or rather: find their way *back*, for that is where all these concepts once had their origin), they encounter there what Heider calls " naïve psychology," "the unformulated or half-formulated knowledge of interpersonal relations as it is expressed in our everyday language and experience" (Heider 1958, 4). As Heider rightly points out, it is this "common-sense psychology" that - more or less influenced by scientific ideas - "guides our behavior toward other people" (and generally in life, one could add). Transferred to psychotherapy, one can and must say: This applies to both sides in the therapeutic relationship, by no means only to the client's side. In their „naïve psychology", therapists are more alike their clients than they sometimes believe.

This is, of course, another challenge to the pursuit of consistency in psychotherapy. On the therapist's side, the theory system of the psychotherapy method she has learned meets a "naïve psychology" already fully formed and quite largely tried and tested in life. "Scientific theory" and "naïve psychology" temporarily enter into a coexistence, in the successful case perhaps a mutual penetration and enrichment in the course of processing inconsistencies between these two. The touchstone for this process will ultimately be the interrelation and the fitting together of the resulting "critical-phenomenal world" of knowledge and half-knowledge, of beliefs and concepts, with the "naïve -phenomenal world" of immediate experience.

The "naïve psychology" of everyday life is so strongly anchored in immediate experience that it outstrips many an intellectually acquired theoretical concept that is incompatible with it in terms of experiential and behavioral effectiveness. One of the strengths of the Gestalt theoretical approach is precisely that it gives priority to phenomenology even in the process of cognition, and thus runs less risk of contradicting people's world of experience in its conceptualizations: "There seems to be a single starting point for psychology, exactly

---

[5] Developed in close cooperation with Beatrice A. Wright. Fritz Heider turns to the analysis of "basic components of our naïve ideas about other people and social situations"; the concepts investigated were "Life space; Perceiving; Causing; Can; Trying; Wanting; Suffering; Sentiments; Belonging; Ought" (1958, 18). The oversimplification of Heider's work in contemporary attribution theories has been countered in recent years primarily by Bertram Malle and his colleagues (Brown University), who also advance Heider's approach in promising ways (Malle 2008, 2011).

as for all the other sciences: the world as we find it, naïvely and uncritically," Wolfgang Köhler says (1947, 3). Even if this is often hard to recognize, the most complex and abstract concepts of the various schools of thought also took their starting point mostly in phenomenology. Henle, to give an example, makes it plausible that Freud's concept of the superego was originally "more a phenomenal report than a psychological theory" (Henle 1962, 398).

Gestalt theory and GTP try to keep this close connection between naïve phenomenology and theoretical-conceptual processing alive and in awareness. This is also an essential basis for mutual understanding in the therapeutic encounter between client and therapist.

From this understanding it also follows for GTP that the therapist's self-experience in her training cannot only be exhausted in working through her own personal history and strivings but must also encompass her own world of ideas and the way she generates these ideas. Therapists often say of themselves, "I'm more the practitioner, not so much the theorist." But this is a big misunderstanding. In fact, there are only practitioners, nothing else: Those practitioners who know something about their implicit theories and thus have an ear for the implicit theories of their clients, and those practitioners who are blind to their own implicit theories and therefore enslaved by them. The latter then also have a hard time being a help to their clients in dealing with the inconsistencies of their world of ideas.

Hilarion G. Petzold expresses a similar, but even more far-reaching thought, when he speaks of the necessity of co-respondence processes in one's own person, the confrontation with the existing 'believe systems' and, on the other hand, of the co-responding, collegial confrontation in the field of research, theory and practice tradition in which one stands" (Petzold 1992, 464).

Alternatives to embedding psychotherapy in an overall theoretical system

To attempt to base the formulation of one's own psychotherapy theory on an overall theoretical system, such as Gestalt theory, is by no means without alternatives. There are also counterarguments. For example, one has pointed out the danger that such an overall system can also tempt one not to take note of facts or possibly even to bend them if they do not fit the chosen system. Festinger's dissonance theory, mentioned above, and related approaches, for example, emphasize this direction unilaterally, without analysis of the concrete conditions that promote or hinder such an erroneous development.

As an alternative to the overall systems, two approaches are mainly advocated today, which partly overlap: on the one hand, eclecticism, the compilation of "evidence-based" techniques and practices without reference to an overarching theory; on the other hand, "overcoming the outdated schools" by integrating different approaches into a „general psychotherapy". We are critical of both approaches - eclecticism for fundamental reasons, but also rash attempts at integration where the conditions for such a general psychotherapy are still lacking.

Mary Henle describes the problem of eclecticism thus: When there are divergent theoretical approaches to a particular topic, it is often the case that neither has a fully satisfactory explanation to offer (otherwise there would be no controversy). "Controversies do not exist in science with regard to processes which are fully understood. Thus, the task seems to be one of arriving at new, more comprehensive theories of the processes in question." (Henle 1957 in 1986, 91) In her view the „parallel between productive solutions of theoretical problems and of personal problems becomes striking", and she refers to C.G. Jung's conviction: "Conflicts are never resolved on their own level. They are outgrown. Only on a higher level can you see both sides." (ibid, 92).

These are also valid arguments in our eyes against a hasty "unification of the schools" in a "general psychotherapy". As desirable as this goal of a new overall system may seem, its achievement cannot be arbitrarily accelerated. Edwin Rausch, eminent German Gestalt psychologist of the second generation, once stated on this subject - referring to the science of psychology:

"While for a later time a development of psychology can be imagined in which the various directions and currents unite, such an integration should not be attempted hastily. In particular, it is to be rejected that one or the other side claims to be able to absorb the Gestalt theory, while in reality its foundations are abandoned or have not been taken note of at all. So it is better to march separately for the time being." (Rausch 1979 in 1992, 144; transl. GSt)

Similarly, Henle has spoken out against a "premature reconciliation of Gestalt psychology and psychoanalysis" (Henle 1986, 85). Such an endeavor needs "a systematic analysis of the assumptions of both psychologies, one concerned with implicit as well as explicit assumptions," to "reveal both important differences and surprising compatibilities of the theories" (86) This is now several decades ago, progress has been made on this path, in many schools of therapy, but it has not yet come to an end. A prerequisite for further progress on this way is the disclosure and reasoning of one's own concepts in their systematic context, not to assert their superiority over all others, but to open them up to scrutiny for similarities and differences. This is also the aim of the presentation of some basic concepts of GTP in this volume.

Petzold's plea for a "plural therapeutic culture" still remains relevant in this state of affairs (Petzold 1992, 460), and will probably remain so in the long run, because - as Kriz puts it - "The diversity of basic concepts thus ultimately reflects the diversity of human life and will therefore always be encountered by us in professional psychotherapy as well..." (Kriz 2014, 15; transl. GSt).

2. Critical Realism: The Epistemic Position of Gestalt Theoretical Psychotherapy

Katharina Sternek[6]

Summary

In this contribution, I discuss the relevance of epistemological models for psychotherapy. Despite its importance epistemology is seldom explicitly dealt within the psychotherapeutic landscape. Based on the presentation of critical realism, the epistemological position of Gestalt Theoretical Psychotherapy (GTP), I intend to show to which extent this explanatory model supports a differentiated understanding of problems between human beings, arising from the differences in experiencing "reality". The presentation deals explicitly with some conclusions that can be drawn from the critical realistic model for practical psychotherapeutic work. In particular, the aspects of basic therapeutic attitude, therapeutic relationship and praxeology are highlighted.

Introduction

In psychotherapy science, there is a certain general emphasis on the demand that psychotherapeutic approaches reveal and reflect the epistemological views that underlie or are inherent in their understanding of psychotherapy, both in their theoretical concepts and their practice (cf. Buchmann, Schlegel & Vetter 1996). In the portrayals of psychotherapeutic methods, however, one rarely finds an explicit response to this claim. As an example, I am referring to an anthology containing the self-presentation of 50 different psychotherapeutic and psychotherapy-related approaches practiced in Austria (Stumm 2011). In his introduction, the editor refers to Petzold's "Tree of Science" (Stumm, 2011a, 13-15) and the necessity that every psychotherapy method must also explicate its basic epistemological assumptions. However, the following descriptions of the various methods in this anthology only in a few cases refer more than peripherally to the epistemological orientation of these various approaches. A similar picture emerges in international compendia (see Corsini & Wedding 2010; Lambert 2013).

If we leave aside those methods and conceptualizations of psychotherapy that do not explicitly deal with their epistemological stance at all, it seems justified to distinguish in the remaining area three main directions of dealing with epistemological questions:

---

[6] Based on a lecture at the 21st Scientific Conference of the GTA "Motion – Spaces of Human Experience," 13th–15th June 2019, Warsaw, Poland, subsequently published in 2021 as an article in a special issue of the e-journal *Gestalt Theory*, 43(1), 13-27, here republished in a revised version.

a. The first of these directions addresses the different "epistemic approaches" people prefer to use to obtain clarity about their situation and possibilities [e.g., "phenomenological, dialectical, empirical-analytical, hermeneutical" (Pieringer & Fazekas 1996, 229ff)] and then determines which of these approaches is addressed primarily and elaborated in a praxeological way in a given therapeutic method. Wagner, for example, ascribes to the Daseinsanalysis a rather phenomenological epistemic process, to modern psychoanalysis a hermeneutical one, to behavioral therapy an empirical-analytical one and to systemic therapy a constructivist one (Wagner, 2007, 169). Against this background and connected to it, there is also a discussion concerning the question of which psychotherapy methods can be effectively integrated with others and which cannot. Buchmann for example, speaks out against a hasty integration of methods which are incompatible in their epistemic approach into a "general psychotherapy", and pleads instead for the explicit presentation and critical reflection of the epistemological positions of the various methods, because: "From these epistemological considerations it seems to be clear that a 'general psychotherapy' that strives for uniformity virtually prevents the further development of psychotherapy." (Buchmann et al. 1996, 108; transl. KS) The same thought is expressed by Norcross & Newman: "Profound epistemological and ontological differences also impede rapid or wholesale integration." (Norcross & Newman 2003, 5) Some heterogeneity of epistemic approaches can also be seen as an opportunity for psychotherapy to develop a "genuine scientific identity" (Slunecko 1996, 294; transl. KS). Alternatively, in more practical terms, "a core skill needed to be an effective therapist is to have developed an awareness of one's own ontological and epistemological positions in relation to one's work as a therapist". (Willig 2019, 1)

b. The second of these directions focuses, above all, on the scope and limitations of human cognition and derives a variety of conclusions from that for many fields of psychotherapy practice. In this regard, the most important example is the debate about (radical) "constructivism" first above all in the community of systemic family therapies (cf. Becvar, 2003), which has also radiated into communities of other therapeutic methods. The "constructivist turn" in the debate among the systemic family therapists has focused on the question of the possibilities of insight and their limitations. The experiential world of human beings is seen as a private construction which consequently must be fully acknowledged by the psychotherapeutic approach, e.g., in founding the therapist's attitude of "impartiality" on this, or in understanding therapy as "a form of conducting a conversation" (Stumm 2011b, 251f; transl. KS), in which the therapist supports the "modification in attribution of meanings." (ibid.)

c. Finally, there is the third direction [to which Gestalt Theoretical Psycho-therapy (GTP) belongs – but probably also to a large extent Petzold's Integrative Therapy], which brings together both previously mentioned directions based on an explicit ontological position (about the human being, human life, the human organism, the human community) and thus bases the entire system of therapy theory and the entire practice on this epistemological position. In this sense, Petzold calls for a consistent scientific approach to method integration in psychotherapy, in which "clarity of the epistemological standpoint" is one of the central criteria (Petzold, 2011, 267). In relation to GTP, Stemberger characterizes this position as follows: "If one compares the therapy theory of GTP with that of other methods, it is striking that in its 'conceptual architecture' the foundation is not a specific praxeology, psychopathology or the like, but a specific epistemological position. This, the so-called critical realism (Köhler, 1968; Bischof, 1966), is the basis for further core concepts of GTP. In GTP, critical realism (CR) is also a fundamental anthropological position – a differentiated statement about man and his world." (Stemberger, 2011, 219f; transl. KS)

Any psychotherapy faces the challenge that besides externally observable behaviors, conditions, and messages of clients, there are obviously "internal processes" that are not directly accessible to the therapist. Psychotherapeutic approaches understand and conceptualize differently this relationship between such an "Inside" and "Outside". From these are drawn representations regarding personality, psychic disorders, as well as appropriate therapeutic treatment. In the following, I shall present the basics of CR, and thereafter consequences will be outlined. The latter ones result from the particular approach for the understanding of human behavior, the therapeutic attitude and therapeutic relationship, as well as praxeology.

Critical Realism

The epistemological position of GTP is based on Critical Realism (CR), as it was formulated first by Köhler 1929; Koffka 1935; Köhler 1938; Metzger 1941 and further elaborated and differentiated by Bischof 1966 and Tholey 1980/2018.

From an ontological angle, Gestalt theory takes a monistic position on the psycho-physical problem (i.e., in simple terms, it advocates the unity of body and soul), but from an epistemological point of view, it takes a dualistic position (Köhler 1971; Tholey 1986/2018). Concerning the epistemological dualism, the central premise of critical realism emphasizes the clear distinction between the transphenomenal world and the phenomenal world. Early experimental results of Gestalt psychology investigated and proved the difference between

23

physical facts and perception, such as Wertheimer "studying the relationship between the organization of the geographical[7] and phenomenal fields." (Luchins & Luchins 1999, 216)

The transphenomenal world encompasses the macrocosm of the physical world and all physical objects and physical organisms which are embedded therein. It is to be understood as the world and a reality that cannot be accessed directly by people. What can be deducted, hypothesized, and said about the transphenomenal world is the interpretation of data obtained with phenomenal means, theoretical constructions, and models. Their data and results constitute the "critical-phenomenal worldview" (Bischof 1966, 28ff) in contrast to the "naïve-phenomenal world" of our everyday life experience. However, within this physical macrocosm, each person (just as every conscious being) has his/her own microcosmic phenomenal world, which he/she perceives and experiences as reality. It is the world that faces every individual and it is intuitively accessible to him/her. The phenomenal world stands for the entire world man experiences: The phenomenally experienced bodily ego and the phenomenal environment which includes the other people.

Based on the distinction of critical realism one speaks of a "doubling of the world" (the concept of epistemological dualism) and one can act on the assumption that the phenomenal world "represents" the transphenomenal world in a more or less adequate way, but not like a "passive image" (it is thus a representational approach to cognition, but one that goes far beyond a mere representational function of consciousness, as will be shown). As Tholey argues (Tholey 1986/2018, 247) this representational effect rather constitutes the end result of a complex process, which can be described as follows: Physical stimuli from the physical environment meet our physical senses and enter (as well as proprioceptive stimuli from the physical body) via afferent neural pathways into the brain to an area in the cerebral cortex, for which Gestalt psychologist Köhler used the term "psychophysical level" (cf. Köhler 1938/1968). At the psychophysical level (PPN) based on physical-physiological processes, a transformation of the stimuli takes place, as a result of which certain contents can be experienced psychologically. In his research, Köhler formulated the so-called "isomorphism assumption." Isomorphism assumes that there is a structural equivalence between physical and physiological processes (brain operations) and psychological operations. This means that for every phenomenon in the

---

[7] The term "geographical" world, which Koffka proposed for the physical macrocosm in 1935, is somewhat misleading according to Metzger, because the science of geography is also part of the phenomenal world (Metzger 2001, 305). For an understanding of the terms "physical", "transphenomenal" and "reality in the first sense" see Walter 2001.

24

experience of the individual there is a corresponding neurophysiological event in the sense of a central nervous counterpart. As a consequence, we have as well to differentiate between our physical organism and our phenomenal bodily ego. Therefore, the question as to why we perceive other persons and objects in front of our perceived bodily ego, could be answered, as Köhler (1929) did.

Concerning the relationship between physical world and phenomenal world, one also assumes a structural equivalence between the physical world and the phenomenal world. "Wertheimer is pointing out that there are resemblances between perception and external world." (Luchins & Luchins 1999, 216) The isomorphism hypothesis, however, can neither be proved nor disproved. I nonetheless would like to mention the debate between Eagle & Wakefield (2007) and Cali (2007) about the relationship of isomorphism with the mirror neuron system. Eagle &Wakefield thereby refer to "historical antecedents" of the idea of isomorphism. (cf. Eagle & Wakefield 2007, 173f) Since the early beginnings of Gestalt psychology several decades ago, the psychophysical approach of critical realism alludes to topics which are recently discussed anew, again in the current discourses of "embodied" and "enacted" cognition. As Clark says, "Human sensing, learning, thought, and feeling are all structured and informed by our body-based interactions with the world around us." (Clark 2012, 275)

From a practical viewpoint, the isomorphism assumption of structural similarity is useful because it explains why human beings are able to move in the physical environment and to interact with this environment, including their fellow human beings, according to their needs. In this sense, the function of the phenomenal world can be regarded as the "steering organ" (cf. Metzger 1986), which supports the orientation of man in the physical world. Elsewhere, I elaborated the following example (see Sternek 2018): While running a man hurts his physical foot by bumping his physical foot against a physical tree root, although he has seen that he has put his experienced foot far from the experienced tree root. The painful feedback shows that there is a difference and mismatch between the position of the physical foot in the physical world and the experienced foot in the experienced world. In our everyday lives, our phenomenal world is generally presented to us as the only real thing – but sometimes, there are experiences that indicate the existence of a transphenomenal world.

The example moreover illustrates the relationship as well between transphenomenal and phenomenal world. It is evident that there exists an interaction between the transphenomenal part of the physical world and the phenomenal part of the physical world. While the physical organism of a person moves in the physical world, his/her phenomenal world is open to influences from the physical/transphenomenal world.

Critical realism also maintains that the phenomenal worlds of human beings are different. Despite the same basic facts in the physical world different experiences emerge in the phenomenal worlds of people. For example: If we hear several persons or eyewitnesses who have observed an automobile accident, we often have a conflict of statements, which normally is not evoked by predilections. This aspect is of particular importance for the psychotherapeutic work, because it supports our knowledge about differences in the perception of situations, which build the base for experience and interpretation of situations and interactions. Many conflicts arising in relationships, for example "who is right" – can be understood as a consequence of the differences within the phenomenal world of people. In the field of psychotherapy, by working with a patient suffering from an eating disorder, who says "I know that I am thin, but I feel thick", Fuchs illustrated in a comprehensible way how useful the critical realistic perspective can be in obtaining an understanding of the patient's view. (Fuchs 2014, 130)

The differences between the phenomenal worlds also arise because the operations in the phenomenal worlds are field events. The phenomenal world is organized as a dynamic field in such a way that all the experience and behavior of the person depends on the field forces between the person and the environment (cf. Lewin 1951). Due to the action of various attractive or repulsive forces, objects in the phenomenal world of a person have a positive or negative character – a "Valenz", which is related to the states of tension determined by personal needs and intentions (see Lindorfer, current volume). In this sense the phenomenological approach of Gestalt Theoretical Psychotherapy is completed by the field-analyses which support our insight for dynamic processes.

However, as we all know, people can speak about their perceptions and their experiences, and they can as well share experiences. As a matter of fact, it is true that despite all the differences between their experiences "their phenomenal worlds [...] are structured by fundamentally similar principles and work in a similar way" (Stemberger 2016, 34; transl. KS). These correspondences in structure and function are the precondition for communication between the individuals and thus form the basic requirement for psychotherapeutic work.

Conclusions for psychotherapeutic work

This epistemological position immunizes Gestalt Theoretical Psychotherapy against a mono-personal view of the human being. GTP as a social and relationship-orientated approach, is characterized by the fact that it regards humans as primarily social beings and not as individuals onto whom social relationships and determinations "are added" only secondarily. Therefore, it also assumes that psychic problems arise in the majority of cases, or indirectly, from troubles in people's social life and their relationships. Some further conclusions that can be drawn from the critical realistic model for practical psychotherapeutic work will now be presented. Firstly, conclusions for the basic psychotherapeutic attitude and for the psychotherapeutic relationship, followed by conclusions concerning praxeology.

Basic attitude of Gestalt-theoretical psychotherapists

Tholey characterizes the basic position of critical realism as follows: "(1) Besides the phenomenal world in which I am, finding things and events, in which I think, feel, make decisions, and communicate with other people who, like me, exist with 'body and soul', there is one transgressive 'transphenomenal' world, which can be subdivided into my physical organism and a physical environment.

(2) In the physical environment are other organisms that have their own phenomenal worlds."(Tholey 1986/2018, 246; transl. KS)

According to Tholey, the acquisition of the second assumption includes "an ethical motive", namely that, if the possibility exists that other beings have a "consciousness", this obliges me to behave in such a way "as if they were consciousness gifted" (ibid).

Since critical realism proceeds from the conviction that a common transphenomenal world exists which is shared with other human beings, this model is linked to ethical demands. To see other people as conscious subjects means that we have to treat them accordingly (Tholey 1986/2018). This requires us to be constantly aware that other people each have their own phenomenal world so that their experience might be different from our own experience. This awareness promotes an attitude of respect for the individual world and the reality of others, especially that of our clients. Because of this attitude, Giuseppe Galli designated the Gestalt theory as a "school of respect" (cf. Galli, 1999, 25). The basic attitudes of respect and objectiveness towards clients indeed characterize GTP. Furthermore, the stance of critical realism is connected to the insight that our actions do not only exist in our phenomenal worlds but also interfere with the transphenomenal world that we share with our fellow human beings, which requires our responsibility.

Psychotherapeutic relationship(s)

Our fundamental conceptualization of the therapeutic relationship, to which a particular effectiveness in psychotherapy is attributed across all schools, is also marked by the critical-realistic perspective.

In a naïve-realistic representation, that is common in everyday life, and as one may read in some conventional psychotherapeutic case presentations, one assumes a therapeutic relationship or situation – that means one therapeutic relationship and one situation. From a critical-realistic point of view, however, as described in detail by Stemberger (2016), there are at least two therapeutic situations: the therapeutic relationship or situation in the phenomenal world of the therapist and the therapeutic relationship or situation in the phenomenal world of the client (Fig.1).

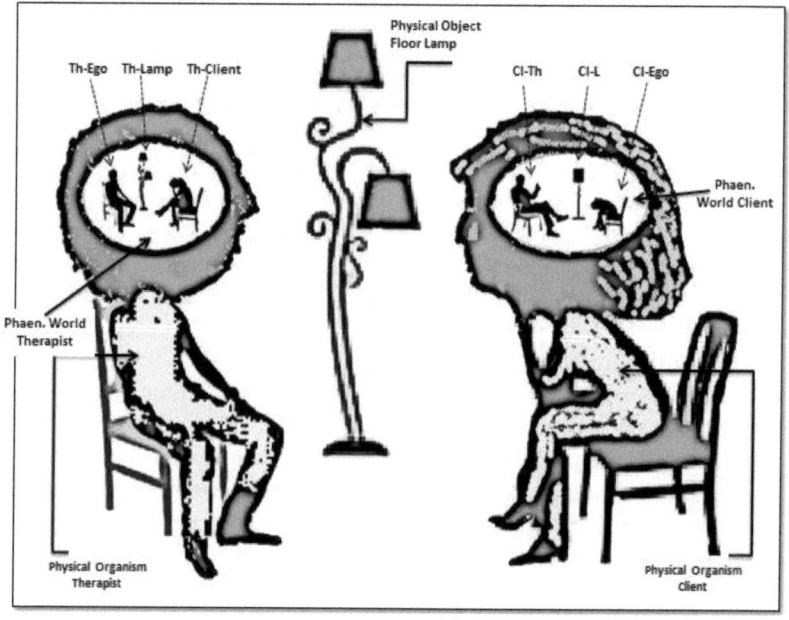

Fig. 1: The therapeutic situation from the critical-realistic perspective (cf. Stemberger 2016, 33) th-ego: phenomenal ego of therapist; th-cl: phenomenal client of the therapist; th-lamp: lamp in the phenomenal world of the therapist.
cl-ego: phenomenal ego of the client; cl-th: phenomenal therapist of the client; cl-lamp: lamp in the phenomenal world of the client

Both the phenomenal world of the therapist and the phenomenal world of the client include one therapist and one client. Stemberger writes: "In the phenomenal world of the client, in this situation, the experienced ego of the client faces his/her phenomenal therapist, and in the phenomenal world of the therapist, the phenomenal ego of the therapist faces his/her phenomenal client."

(Stemberger 2016, 33; transl. KS) This approach is constitutive for the entire therapeutic process. Accordingly, a permanent readiness is required for mutual exchange between client and therapist about their reciprocal experience – not one restricted to conflict between the parties. Although both are in a common transphenomenal world and therefore interact with each other, they sometimes experience events in psychotherapy very differently. Therefore, the therapist needs to be aware of these differences. An awareness of these differences should support him/her to reflect critically his/her own perception of the therapeutic relationship, in combination with the awareness to be mistaken regarding the quality of this relationship.

Considering the eminent importance of the therapeutic relationship for the success or failure of psychotherapeutic work, a further question is central: How do I as therapist appear and act in the phenomenal world of the client, that is, how am I experienced by the client (as a supportive therapist, as a critical or judging therapist, as a comforting therapist, …). Conversely, just as important too is the question how the client appears in my phenomenal world (as a difficult, acting client, as a client who puts a lot of strain on me, as a client who annoys me, or as an admiring client, …). According to the critical realistic standpoint of GTP, this question cannot only be answered by the concept of transference or countertransference (cf. Kästl 2007).

In summary, the critical realistic perspective thus shapes the overall attitude of the therapist in his/her interaction with the client. It contributes to promote an attitude of the therapist, to critically deal with his/her own experience and evaluation of the therapeutic relationship and the therapeutic situation, followed by an effort for open, transparent, communication and mutual coordination. As language plays an important role within communication, therapists should train their sensitivity for language, especially for "double meaning of hybrid terms and shift-of-situations." (cf. Buchholz 2020, 127).

At least, adequately internalized, the critical realistic perspective and the associated basic attitude may represent protection for the therapeutic relationship: It protects the client's dignity as her/his experience is encountered with respect. Furthermore, it protects the client from the alleged superiority of the therapist and the therapist from being seduced by fantasies of omnipotence. In contrast to some asymmetry that could arise with a particular comprehension of the roles of client and therapist – on the one hand, a client who sees himself/herself as seeking help, and on the other hand, a therapist who imagines himself to be allocated a special power ostensibly resulting from the deemed sovereignty of interpretation which is, by default, assigned to therapists by reason of the subjective nature of psychotherapeutic practice, transparent interactions between therapist and client can counteract the reinforcement of imaginary hierarchies of power, as well as their narcissistic abuse.

Praxeology

Consequently, the critical realistic approach exerts influence on the praxeology: A centerpiece of praxeology of GTP is the phenomenological approach, followed and completed by the field analysis. (see Stemberger 2016)

When we talk about the therapist "practicing phenomenology together with his client", we mean that the therapist encourages his client to take his own phenomenal world seriously. The therapist promotes the client to explore his/her phenomenal world, which is a world with field character (wherein attractive and repulsive field forces are effective) not only with the help of logical reasoning, but with all his/her senses in order to support the client to clarify his/her situation and possibilities for action.

In the context of his field theory, Kurt Lewin writes that this is a genuinely psychological approach: "One of the basic characteristics of field theory in psychology, as I see it, is the demand that the field which influences an individual should be described not in 'objective physicalistic' terms, but in the way in which it exists for that person at that time."(Lewin 1951a, 62)

Lewin even emphasizes: "A teacher will never succeed in giving proper guidance to a child if he does not learn to understand the psychological world in which that individual child lives. To describe a situation 'objectively' in psychology actually means to describe the situation as a totality of those facts and of only those facts which make up the field of that individual. To substitute for that world of the individual the world of the teacher, of the physicist, or of anybody else is to be, not objective, but wrong." (ibid.)

In this context, Lewin agrees with critical realism to the extent to Koffka's distinction between the "behavioral environment" of man and his "geographical environment" (cf. Koffka 1935, 27f). As early as 1935, Koffka demonstrates with the story "The ride over the Lake of Constance" that experience and behavior of a human being are determined by the behavioral environment (phenomenal world) and not by the "geographical", physical environment.

GTP too confirms that the individually experienced world is a decisive factor in determination of the client's experience and behavior. Therefore, within the psychotherapeutic work, we focus our questions and interventions on the analyses of the phenomenal world. As a consequence of the therapist's psychotherapeutic work, a change of centering (see Fuchs, current volume) in the phenomenal world of the client can happen in such a way that he/she is enabled to solve his/her problems. Therefore, "practicing phenomenology" means to jointly explore the client's phenomenal world; to be more precise: it involves supporting the client in exploring her/his phenomenal world, since the latter is not imminently accessible to the therapist, but only indirectly through the constant exchange with the client. During the therapeutic process, the therapist – monitoring his/her phenomenal perspective to try to understand the client and to notice inconsistency and contrariness – can offer his/her perspective to the client to the extent that it supports the client's development.

The Gestalt psychologist Metzger described several differentiations within the phenomenal world. The most important differentiation for the practical therapeutic work is the following one: Regarding the immediate experience Metzger discriminates between what is directly encountered, bodily encountered and facing us, and what is brought to mind, thought, suspected, remembered, planned, constructed, conceptualized, or expected (cf. Metzger 2001, 8-47).

Indeed, some former Lewin students (Brown 1933; Mahler 1933) have demonstrated in various studies that what is experienced in the direct encounter is "more real", and in many cases more effective, for behavior than the merely thought of or visualized experience. For example: It makes a huge difference to a person, whether he/she knows intellectually that his/her fear can be traced back to the memory of certain past or future events or whether he/she encounters that fear directly in his/her experience. One consequence which falls within the scope of our psychotherapeutic work is that we can assist our client to face his/her fear in "the here and now", not only by talking about it, but also by processing and overcoming it within a setting of supporting conditions and interventions.

In our psychotherapeutic work we use the knowledge about Metzger's distinction by offering experience-centered interventions (e.g., working with the empty chair, body awareness exercises), as long as we intend to support the client to get in contact with his/her immediate experience. For example, working with the empty chair can enable clients to empathize with the encountered other and to experience how the other feels. At best, the client gains more insight into the dynamic of the motives and the relation. However, there are also circumstances in which the opposite of direct confrontation is required, such as working with traumatized people who suffer from flashbacks or intrusive memories. These cases require targeted interventions that help those affected to obtain a greater distance from their immediate experience [e.g., screen-technic (see Sternek 2014)]. The essential advantage of a clear distinction is therefore – if the therapist notices what is at stake – the clarity with which the choice for appropriate interventions is exercised.

However, this does not mean that in GTP no importance is attached to the world of thoughts, ideas, the known and the believed. There is rarely, if ever, an immediate perception that is not consciously or non-consciously influenced by ideas and concepts (whether scientifically based or not). Further differentiation is therefore important, namely Bischof's distinction between the naïve-phenomenal and the critical-phenomenal world (cf. Bischof 1966, 28ff.). For Bischof, the naïve-phenomenal world refers to the perceptual world of everyday experience, that is, the experienced bodily ego and experienced environment. In contrast, the critical-phenomenal world encompasses all known facts, research findings, and assumptions regarding the body schema, the world schema, the organism, the physical world, etc., whether these are scientific insights or everyday assumptions of lay people. Stemberger points out that "all own explanations for the relationship in the world belong to the critical-phenomenal world, ... all beliefs, convictions and ideologies, including all related problems, doubts, and pricks of consciences." (Stemberger 2016, 32; transl. KS)

As psychotherapists, we sometimes meet clients who suffer from problems which are predominantly based on fixed assumptions. For example, one female client, who wishes to have a satisfying partnership, which does not happen, says: "I know that at least all guys are liars who use their phrases only to impress women. But in fact, they have simply one thing in mind, to manipulate and use women". This basic conviction then – in the sense of a "naïve theory" (cf. Heider 1958) – influences the experience and behavior of the person concerned. As there is a mutual influence or superposition of the naïve -phenomenal world and the critical-phenomenal world, such a "theory about the nature of male human beings" contributes under certain circumstances that particular problems arise in the first place and inhibits their solution. In the light of her "theory" about man, the woman in our example cannot really meet a man without distrust and prejudice. In such and similar cases, psychotherapeutic work can not only deal with the naïve-phenomenal world and the experience of a human being, but must also address his (or her) self-assumed convictions and explanatory models.

Accordingly, the non-observance or neglect of everyday explanations of our clients would appear as an omission. One must not refuse all of this with arguments like intellectualism or rationalism. To do justice to our clients in psychotherapy, the "practicing of phenomenology" (Stemberger 2016, 34f) necessitates the inclusion of both the critical-phenomenal world as well as the naïve-phenomenal world of the client. As psychotherapists, we should be encouraged to reflect on the question of whether and how far our beliefs and theories may unconsciously influence our perception, evaluation, and behavior. At this point I fully agree with Willig's demand that "a core skill needed to be an effective therapist is to have developed an awareness of one's own ontological and epistemological position in relation to one's work as a therapist." (Willig

2019, 1) Furthermore, in general, it seems to be clear that similarity of the basic assumptions of the therapist and the client support the understanding of a client's distress (ibid.). But there is one point in which I differ from Willig's claim "that client and therapist share assumptions about the nature of human being and experiencing" (ibid., 2), because within the mutual exchange, the difference, if it is not too radical, could also be regarded as conducive for the therapeutic process.

Finally, some short comment concerning diagnosis needs to be mentioned. The critical realistic perspective can protect against acceptance of diagnostic classification that is based on a pragmatic agreement or on an ultimately untenable self-conception about reality. Our clients derive little benefit of such a classification. On the contrary – classifications can imply that we no longer consider some things to be worthy of clarification. (cf. Beneder 2015). Therefore, the critical realistic approach can support us to meet our clients in as unbiased a manner as possible.

Final remark

The epistemological position of critical realism offers an explanatory model of how differences in the perception and the experience of people arise, and thereafter also conflicts. This epistemological background is useful because it contributes to a better understanding of dynamic interactions in social relationships. Hence, it supports the formation of a constructive relationship in the field of psychotherapy and in all other areas in which people try to constructively support each other. Several tasks are connected to this objective, in particular the aim of doing justice to the clients who have entrusted themselves to the care of the psychotherapist to bring about an improvement in their reality of life and experience, and this is not in the least a question of the prerequisites and possibilities of our knowledge. Finally, it should be comprehensible that the system of therapeutic theory and practice of GTP achieves the demand of being based on a clear epistemological position.

3. Personality Theory in Gestalt Theoretical Psychotherapy: Kurt Lewin's Field Theory and Theory of Systems in Tension Revisited

Bernadette Lindorfer[89]

Summary

   With regard to the dynamics of human experience and behavior, Gestalt Theoretical Psychotherapy (GTP) is mainly based on Kurt Lewin's dynamic field theory of personality. GTP is carried out by including a re-interpretation of Lewin's theory in some aspects of psychotherapeutic practice on basis of critical realism. Human experience and behavior are understood to be functions of the person and the environment (including the other individuals therein) in a psychic field (life space), which encompasses both of these mutually dependent factors. The anthropological model of this approach is, therefore, not mono-personal but, a priori, structural and relational in nature. It does not one-sidedly focus on the "inner components" of a person, but on the interrelation between the individual and a given environment, which affects experience and behavior. After a brief introduction of these basic concepts, this lecture will focus especially on Lewin's concept of tension systems, which may be considered as the Gestalt theoretical counterpart of Freud's drive theory. Further, we define the basic assumptions which underlie GTP and explain how the person moves through her/his life experience in terms of Gestalt psychology.

1. Introduction

   Psychotherapy is an intentional, planned, interactional process that implies that the therapist has assumptions about the human person and its functioning and about the nature and functioning of such an interactional process. Whether explicit or implicit, naïve or scientific, every psychotherapist has some kind of personality " theory" (at least a set of assumptions, which does not have to be either systematic or without contradictions) that is involved in guiding her/his actions. One can understand a client's anxiety as a punishment from God, an innate constitutional trait, a learned reaction, an expression of unresolved instinctual conflicts, or as a result of the client's psychological situation. Depending on her/his assumptions – whether or not she/he is aware of them – the therapist will experience the situation differently and will interact differently with the client. Since psychotherapy schools

[8] Based on a lecture at the 21st Scientific Conference of the GTA "Motion – Spaces of Human Experience," 13th–15th June 2019, Warsaw, Poland, subsequently published in 2021 as an article in a special issue of the e-journal *Gestalt Theory*, 43(1), 13-27, here republished in a revised version.

[9] I am very grateful to Gerhard Stemberger for initiating this contribution and for supporting and advising on its creation with great knowledge and prudence.

consider themselves to be scientific, they are subject to the requirement to make explicit assumptions, and thus also render these debatable and verifiable. By also reflecting on their own implicit, naïve, and prescientific personality conceptions, therapists improve their ability to recognize and understand the naïve "personality theories" that underlie their clients' experiences.

Scientific personality theories intend to describe, explain, and predict the individual peculiarities in the way people experience themselves and their world and behave in it. Usually, these theories include terms and concepts about personality structure, its dynamics and development. To date, no consensual paradigm exists, but there are many different approaches in academic psychology and in the field of psychotherapy. According to an earlier "classic" in this field, Hall and Lindzey (1978), originally there were two main lines of personality theories, one emanating from the clinical area, from Gestalt psychology and the works of William Stern, and the other from empirical, natural science-oriented psychology. Since then, these lines have further differentiated: some new ones have been added, some habe lost importance. However, a fundamental dividing line between the more holistic-oriented approaches from the clinical area and the behavioral, trait-oriented, factor-analytical, and biological (genetic and neurobiological) approaches of academic psychology have remained noticeable (e.g., Weiner, Millon, & Lerner 2003; Corr & Matthews 2009).

Kurt Lewin's holistic, Gestalt-, and field-oriented personality theory had a high influence on the emerging personality psychology. It moved away from the prevailing static models of personality in favor of a dynamic one. Behavior is no longer seen as a manifestation of character or of traits, but as a functional part of the situation (Foschi & Lombardo 2006). Contrary to his initially great influence, interest in Lewin's concept of personality decreased at the end of the 20th century in the field of academic personality psychology. Thus, his ideas are presented in the two-volume overview work by Hall & Lindzey until the 1978 edition but were no longer included in later editions. In contrast, other humanistic approaches and neo-psychoanalytic approaches are given more importance. Likewise, other recent publications on personality theories in academic psychology no longer deal explicitly with Kurt Lewin's field approach, although often the traces of his ideas and concepts are unmistakable even where his name is not mentioned.

Various approaches that were developed in the framework of Lewin's field theory are still being pursued today without explicitly placing them in the context of a personality theory. For example, Lewin's theory of systems in tension occupies a prominent place in Heinz Heckhausen's standard work Motivation and Action (Heckhausen 1991, 113–127) and continues to do so in the revised third edition (2018), which was published after Heckhausen's death and in which his concept is contrasted with other models (Heckhausen & Beckmann 2018).[10] Lewin's theory of systems in tension also underlies the still unbroken series of experimental research on the resumption of interrupted actions as well as the development of newer theories based on it, such as the concept of symbolic self-completion by Wicklund and Gollwitzer (1981, 1982) and the approaches that emerged from it.

A continuation of Lewin's ideas in the field of cognitive psychology comes from Rainio (2009), His "Discrete Process Model" draws substantially on the ideas of Lewin, which he considers as a "very good basis for modern holistic theory of cognition and behavior". Finally, Duch (2017), by recourse to Rainio's "Discrete Process Model" tries to make Lewin's field theory of personality fruitful in the domain of neurophysiology and neuropsychology by relating the dynamic field theory of the person to the dynamics of brain processes – something Lewin himself considered as negligible with regard to psychological theory, but which was especially emphasized and conceptualized in Gestalt theory by Köhler (1968; see also section 2).

Summarizing so far, there seems to be a difference between the requirements for a personality theory in academic psychology and the requirements for one in psychotherapy. In academic psychology, the necessity and possibility of a personality theory can be assessed sometimes more and sometimes less highly in the course of the development of psychology. In psychotherapy, on the other hand, the entire therapeutic methodology depends on one's own ideas about personality and its functioning, and the concepts are put to the test day after day. It is therefore not surprising that Lewin's field theory and his suggestions for understanding the person still play an important role in the field of psychotherapeutic theories and concepts. This is the case, for example, with group therapy methods, with group psychoanalysis (Foulkes, Bion) and system-centered therapy for groups by Yvonne M. Agazarian (1986, 2004), with the conditional genetic psychopathology of the catathymic-imaginative approach of H.C. Leuner (1997; Andersch 2012), with Gestalt therapy (Wollants 2008; Staemmler 2005; Spagnuolo-Lobb 2010), and with the more recent field-theoretical approaches in psychoanalysis (Baranger & Baranger 2008).

---

[10] However, a possible contradiction between a "person model" (to which the systems in tensions are assigned) and an "environment model" (in which the valences in the environment play a central role) is suspected in Lewin's field theory by the authors, an assessment we do not follow.

This article aims to show how Kurt Lewin's concept of personality is understood and embedded in the theoretical framework of Gestalt Theoretical Psychotherapy and how it is put into practice there.

2. Gestalt Theory as Field Theory

For Gestalt theory and Gestalt Theoretical Psychotherapy, the epistemological viewpoint of critical realism, and thus the strict distinction between the phenomenal and the transphenomenal world and the specific understanding of the nature and function of the relations between these worlds, is crucial (Köhler 1929; Bischof 1966; Metzger 1969; Stemberger 2011; Sternek 2021). The interrelation between the transphenomenal world and the phenomenal world is assumed to be isomorphic (Köhler 1968; Luchins & Luchins 1999). Gestalt theory is a field theory per se (Metzger 1975 in 1986, 220). According to Tholey (1998) and Stemberger (2019), we can distinguish between the phenomenal field, the psychic field, and the psychophysical field. These differentiations have also important implications for psychotherapy. The phenomenal field includes the phenomenal bodily ego and its phenomenal environment. It is the everyday world of human experience, that we address mainly when we are "practicing phenomenology" with our clients. It is the world "in which we perceive, think, remember, plan, act, communicate, and interact" (ibid., 62). Extended by the (psychological) forces that are phenomenally not given but show themselves through their action or effects – for example, Prägnanz tendency, frame of reference, and so on as quasi-phenomenal constructs in the field of Gestalt theory, or the id and the unconscious forces of defense or resistance as constructs in the field of depth psychology – it becomes a psychic/psychological field. The third, psychophysical field is a postulated central nervous field, which is simultaneously psychic and physical. In this respect, this concept contains the Gestalt theoretical idea that mental processes are that part of the totality of central nervous processes which also has phenomenal properties and constitutes consciousness. It differs significantly from parallelistic theories and approaches that attribute a causal relationship – in terms of cause and effect – between central nervous and psychological processes, the psyche, and the brain.

Lewin's field approach, which is fundamental for the personality theory in Gestalt Theoretical Psychotherapy, deals with the psychological field. In GTP, Lewin's approach is consistently interpreted in a critical-realistic way, which in some areas leads to different results than those available in the writings of Lewin himself. As is well known, Kurt Lewin differed from the other founders of Gestalt theory in one essential point, namely, the necessity of a psychophysical theory, as proposed by Wertheimer, Köhler, and Koffka.

This led to problems in Lewin's central concept of life space, whose relationship to the non-psychological environment of the life space remained contradictory in Lewin's work (Graefe presented a detailed study of this problem in 1961). However, these contradictions can be resolved on a critical-realistic basis, which is now consistently carried out in the conceptualization of GTP. Without a solution to this problem, it would not be possible to adequately understand and treat the processes of people's encounters and relationships in psychotherapy, because here (as in everyday situations where people interact) not one but several life spaces come into play, and it is therefore necessary to understand how the mutual influences between these life spaces come about.[11] Contrary to Lewin's view, this makes a psycho-physical theory inevitable.

In other words, in Gestalt theoretical psychotherapy, the understanding of the experience and behavior of client and psychotherapist, as well as all other subconcepts of our psychotherapy conception, are consequently based on the field-theoretical approach of Gestalt theory: Nevertheless, we are convinced that such a field theory has to be a psychophysical one (with the "discovery" of the "4Es" this view has meanwhile also gained attention in the cognitive sciences). In this respect, our concepts are built on the fruitful notions and findings of Lewin's field theory, but they do not follow its limitation to a purely psychological field theory. Instead, Gestalt Theoretical Psychotherapy integrates Lewin's concepts and findings into the general psychophysical field theory of the Gestalt theoretical approach, for which Köhler's isomorphism assumption is still the most plausible hypothesis regarding the relationship between psychological and physical processes.

3. Lewin's Field Theory

3.1. The concept of life space

It was Lewin's scientific claim not to be satisfied with general laws about generalized people, but to develop a terminology that allows one to explain the single case and to answer the question of why in a particular case a given individual behaves in a given way and not otherwise (Lewin 1936, 11). Therefore, Lewin argues, we have to know the laws which control psychological events – for example, the dynamic laws in the field of needs and emotions – and the specific nature of the particular situation the person is placed in. Hence, the focus of investigation in Lewin's theory is the person-in-a-situation, which is called "life space." The life space with the person and her/his

---

[11] Paul Tholey has pointed out that this problem has been underestimated in the initial publications on Gestalt Theoretical Psychotherapy (Tholey 1996, 11f)

psychological environment is seen as a dynamic field that is continuously changing and encompasses everything that determines the person's experience and behavior at a given time.

The environment and the person are further articulated into "regions." The person is seen as a stratified system with central and peripheral regions. The regions of the environment are the quasi-social, quasi-physical, and quasi-conceptual facts that we find therein. Regions are qualitatively different from each other and are separated by boundaries, which are more or less permeable. For our experience and behavior, it is of great importance in which way and to what degree these regions are connected or separated (Lewin 1936, 42).

Not all regions of the life space are equally accessible to the person. We often find bodily, physical, social, or mental boundaries that prevent us from locomotion to a special region. Yet, the solidity of the boundaries can be different with respect to the specific (bodily, social, or mental) sphere. Besides all kinds of physical, social, or mental barriers, the zone of free movement is limited by insufficient (physical or mental) ability (Lewin 1936, 45). In order to understand or even predict a person's behavior, it is therefore essential to determine his/her location in the life space.

Our environment includes many objects and events having specific characteristics for us: some invite us to eat or drink them, some can protect us against cold or rain, another lures us to play with it, this relaxed person seems able to calm us down, that lively person to cheer us up ... The objects and events have a special "valence," as Lewin says, which is a "stimulating character" that invites us to act. Depending on our current goals and needs and the associated tension systems (see chapter 4), this valence can be positive or negative and varies in its strength (Lewin 1935; Lück 1996). So, when I am hungry, the bakery will catch my eye, while I do not notice the hairdresser's next to it. If I have next day's job interview in mind, the hairdresser gets my attention and calls me in – now the bakery doesn't mean anything to me and I may not even notice it. Needs and goals and the resulting valences do not always emanate from the person. They can also arise from the environment and can be induced especially by other persons and groups but also by environmental facts or events and their power fields.

Because it is a field, the facts in the life space (objects, persons, activities) are related to each other and the person and the environment must be regarded as being mutually interdependent. If and how an object, person, or event is experienced in our phenomenal world is therefore a result of a dynamic process of organization, in which at first the Gestalt properties of the object or event and the total configuration in the perceptual field play a substantial role. Furthermore, this field is in close communication with the overall "inner" situation, especially the prevailing goals, intentions, and needs (cf. Soff 2018). Therefore, there is a direct relationship between the momentary state of the individual and the structure of her/his psychological environment.

In this view, behavior is the result of change in some state of the field in a given unit of time. Behavior in Lewin's field concept depends neither on the past nor on the future, but on the present field in the "here and now." Indubitably, of course, the present field has a certain time depth that includes both the psychological past and the psychological future with its expectations, wishes, and dreams (Lewin 1936; 1942).[12]

The life space develops and changes during our entire life. As the individual matures and develops, the life space expands and its differentiation increases. Some regions become accessible, others inaccessible, and the valences of regions are, perhaps, changing.

3.2. The concept of forces

However, the state of intentions, needs, and goals of the person on the one hand, and the valences of objects and activities on the other hand do not determine sufficiently what behavior will occur. Thus, Lewin uses the concept of force. He postulates that all experience and behavior depend on the field forces that are operational between the person and his/her psychological environment. Forces are defined by their direction, their strength, and their point of application; and they are represented by vectors. To put it briefly, driving-field forces that correspond with positive valences cause us to move toward a goal or object, and field forces corresponding with negative valences cause us to move away from it. This is not only meant in a physical sense but also in a figurative sense. Barriers in the life space that prevent us from attaining a goal correspond to restraining forces. The totality of the forces present in the psychological field will control the direction of the process and thus the behavior (Lewin 1946/1963).

In this process, we often meet conflicting forces. Therefore, we often have to pass a region with a negative valence to reach our goal, as when we first have to go through exams before we get permission to work in a specific profession, or when we have to do boring and monotonous exercises before we become good at something. Sometimes, we are torn between two approximately equally attractive alternatives. However, since the balance is rather unstable, we are unlikely to remain trapped in this conflict for long. An

---

[12] Lewin's 1942 publication "Time perspective and morale" is considered the foundation of psychological theory and research on time perspective. For some recent work on the psychological time depth, see Nuttin, J. & W. Lens (1985); Stolarski, M., N. Fieulaine & W. van Beek (eds., 2015) and Zimbardo, P.C. & J.N. Boyd (1999).

approach in the direction of one of the alternatives soon will lead to its predominance over the other. In other situations, we find, simultaneously, attraction and repulsion in the same place; consequently, at a certain point, there may be hesitation, a halt, or a back-and-forth movement in the approach to the goal.

Where the attainment of a goal is impeded by some barrier, the action toward the goal will not completely stop. It will initially push the action out of the original direction. However, if the individual runs against the barrier several times without success, the barrier itself acquires a negative valence. In addition to a positive vector, a negative one comes into existence.

When conflicts become very strong, it can sometimes happen that the individual no longer faces the conflict but "goes out of the field"; this can be physical again, but may also occur as resignation, inner emigration, etc. In every process, the forces in the inner and outer environment are changed by the process itself (Lewin 1935, 48).

4. Lewin's Theory of Systems in Tension

Up to this point we focused mainly on the interaction between the person and the environment and the associated forces in the life space. Now we will turn more closely to the area of the person, especially to the sphere of the person's needs, intentions, and goals, which is essential to the dynamics of the mind.

We know that every process that takes place presupposes energy that is set free and capable of doing the work – but where do these energies come from?

Kurt Lewin worked on this issue in Berlin as early as the 1920s. In his publications, "Vorbemerkungen über die psychischen Kräfte und Energien und über die Struktur der Seele" [Preliminary Remarks on the Psychological Forces and Energies and on the Structure of the Mind] (1926a) and "Vorsatz, Wille und Bedürfnis [Intention, Will, and Need]," (1926b), he formulated his fundamental ideas. At the same time, together with his co-workers and students, he began to carry out a series of investigations to test these theses experimentally. The results were published between 1926 and 1937 in about 20 articles, mainly in the journal "Psychologische Forschung" [Psychological Research].

In short, Lewin assumes that the energies required for behavior are to be found in psychic tensions that arise when there is a need, a wish, a purpose, or an intention. The latter are called "quasi-needs." These psychic tensions are striving for discharge and thus make us ready for action: "The inner state of tension comes to a breakthrough as soon as the possibility of eliminating or at least alleviating the tension seems to exist, i.e., as soon as there is a situation in which one senses the possibility of actions in the direction of the goal" (Lewin 1926b, 349; translation BL). Once the need has been satisfied or the goal has been achieved, the tension lessens and the system finds a new equilibrium. This is the same, whether the tension stems from a genuine need, a quasi-need, or a need which is induced by the power field of another person, group, or institution – they are functionally identical. Equally, the fulfillment of a given need leads to the release of the tension and a reestablishment of an equilibrium (Lewin 1926b; Brown 1929; Marrow 1969, 33).

Here we find some significant differences between Lewin's motivation theory and instinct or drive theories as Freud's. Lewin's concept is open to all sorts of motivational needs: not only basic bodily needs such as hunger, thirst, and sexuality but also essential mental and social needs, for example, social bonding, self-esteem, belonging, curiosity, self-efficacy, self-esteem, and others. Quasi-needs, i.e., intentions, purposes, goals, and wishes, often derive from them and are in a close dynamic communication with them. Both needs and quasi-needs develop and change throughout life, and social factors and relationships play an important role in this. Thus, they can arise from altruistic motivation (an action is performed for the sake of another person), can be induced by the power field of another person or group ("induced needs"), or emerge from the state of belonging to a group and the desire to share and follow its goals (Lewin 1946/1963).

This has manifold implications for psychotherapy. So, it will be important to clarify with the client whether her/his behavior arises from her/his own needs and intentions or is induced by the power field of other persons or groups, which can be experienced either as supportive or restrictive (cf. Lindorfer, 2017). Related to this, the question of how the client can develop and strengthen her/his power field is of particular importance. Further, the success of the therapist-client joint effort in psychotherapy will also depend on the extent to which the therapist can develop and flexibly use her/his power field toward the client (cf. Stemberger 2017a,b)[13.]

In contrast to Lewin's conceptualization, drive theories mostly view the motivations underlying behavior as innate or inherent, arising in development. They are usually understood as continuously acting in a certain direction. However, Lewin underlines that the efficacy of the drives is bound to the existence of acute states of tension (Lewin 1928).

---

13 In the view of critical realism we have to differentiate between the therapeutic relationship in the phenomenal world of the psychotherapist and the therapeutic relationship in the phenomenal world of the client (see section 7, also Böhm in this volume). In the context here, we refer to the power field in the client's phenomenal world.

Mostly – and maybe also on the basis of Freud's view that we strive for pleasure and avoid displeasure – the term "tension" is used to describe an unpleasant state of strain or stress; but this is not what Lewin meant by the term. According to his concept, "tension" is, rather, a desirable state because it is valuable for increasing a person's efforts to achieve a goal (cf. Marrow 1969, 31f).

5. Experimental Work of the Lewin Group on Tension Systems

From the beginning Gestalt theory has advocated an experimental approach. Contrary to the usual investigations up to that time, experiments based on Gestalt theory were supposed to do justice to the holistic nature of mental processes and to aim at results that would make a difference in life practice. Accordingly, Lewin and his co-workers also set out to further develop and verify his dynamic theory of personality by experimental means.

5.1. Forgetting and remembering

The basic experimental verification of Lewin's concept was carried out by Bluma Zeigarnik (1927) and Maria [Rickers-]Ovsiankina (1928/1976). Both deal with the tensions arising from taking on a task. Zeigarnik presented the subjects a number of tasks (22) to perform. The tasks were of all kinds and levels of difficulty, and included, for example, the continuation of a honeycomb pattern, disentangling puzzle-rings, guesswork, laying mosaics of colored stones, solving jigsaw puzzles, threading pearls on a string, memory tests, etc. While the subjects were allowed to finish half of the tasks, they were interrupted in the other half by the presentation of a new task at a time when they were well on the way to a solution. The subjects of course didn't know whether or why they would be allowed to complete a task or not. At the end of the session, the experimenter asked them to tell her what they had been doing during the hour. On average the unfinished tasks were recalled twice as often as the completed tasks.

After Bluma Zeigarnik proved wrong some other possible explanations for these results (emotional shock by the interruption; did subjects expect to be asked later to complete the tasks?), she concluded that we must find the cause of the better recollection of the uncompleted tasks in the tension set up by the intended act, which corresponds to a quasi-need:

The question of the experimenter "What have you been doing in this hour?" sets up a tension in the subject that will be relieved by the recall. Similarly, each task in the experiment had also set up a tension that was discharged when the task was completed, but remained unrelieved for the interrupted tasks. Therefore, at the moment of recall, two vectors exist, deriving from these two tensions: one driving in direction of the recall of all the tasks, the other directed toward the completion of the unfinished tasks. The latter becomes effective also for the recall, making the unfinished tasks more readily available.

Bluma Zeigarnik's experiment was a first proof of the validity of Lewin's concept of psychic tension. It became very popular, and many follow-up studies were carried out. Its results were confirmed in most cases but couldn't always be replicated. This led to a refined understanding of the phenomenon. Hence, there is no evidence for an autonomous need to complete something we have started. The extent of retention is dependent on how committed we were to the task and whether the mastery of the task affected such central personal goals as, for example, our self-esteem. When the subjects' ambition is aroused, the number of uncompleted tasks at the recall grows enormously.

Furthermore, the expectations of the subjects have a significant impact on what will become figure and what will become ground. If my level of aspiration and my self-esteem are low, I will probably better recall the completed tasks, whereas someone whose self-esteem and level of aspiration are high is better in the recall of the unfinished tasks (Junker 1960).

Another important finding of Zeigarnik was that tensions are not set up unless there is a certain stability in the total psychic field. In cases of fatigue and excitability, no tensions are established. As a result of subsequent emotional upsets, existing tension systems can be destroyed.

After a certain time – a few days or so – tensions that stem from the unresolved tasks may disappear naturally (cf. Lindorfer 2012a).

5.2. Resumption and completion

If a purpose or an intention corresponds dynamically to a tension system, it is to be expected that once set up, it will not just affect memory but will also cause activities which serve the purpose of execution. This assumption was examined by Maria [Rickers-]Ovsiankina (1928/1976), another student of Lewin. Similarly to Zeigarnik's experiments, the subjects were given different tasks and were interrupted in some of their activities. After a while, they were left alone in the room.

Ovsiankina discovered a natural tendency toward resumption. The vast majority of the subjects returned to the uncompleted activities to finish them off. When the experimenter forbade resumption, resumption of an underhand nature occurred. However, once an activity was completed and the goal was achieved, resumption failed to occur. Instead, there was relaxation, satisfaction, and an indifference to the task. The decisive factor here was the achievement of the inner and not the outer goal of the action. In accordance with Zeigarnik's findings, the tendency for resumption in [Rickers-]Ovsiankina's study depended essentially on the subjects attitudes toward the action. The more the subject got involved in the task, the more likely they were to resume. Highest resumption rates occured when the person devoted herself / himself to the task with "dedication." Again, ambition increases the frequency of resumption. In both cases, strong needs are addressed (cf. Lindorfer 2012b).

5.3. Substitution: completion by replacement

What happens if an action is interrupted and there is no way to resume and complete it? What happens to the tension then? What happens when the original inner goal of action can no longer be achieved? How can a conclusion be found in this case? These are the questions that Lewin's co-workers Lissner (1933), Mahler (1933), and Sliosberg (1934) investigated in their experiments.

Käte Lissner (1933) also used the technique of interrupted tasks to examine which sort of substitute actions could release the built-up tension systems and so prevent the interrupted actions from being resumed. The extent to which the tendency to resume was reduced was defined as "substitute value." The factors "similarity" and "difficulty" turned out to be essential. Specifically, the similarity to the inner goal of the action is decisive and not the external similarity of the action. In addition, under identical circumstances, the more difficult action had a higher substitute value.

Wera Mahler's study (1933) revealed that substitute actions with a higher degree of reality are of more value than those with a lower degree. Hence, a substitute action is more likely to discharge the tension than a substitution by talking. Again, it is crucial to understand whether the person's inner goal is achieved. Thus, communicating a solution for a problem-task can already be a kind of realization, because it is creating a social fact, but doing so in implementation tasks – such as building a tower – is not sufficient.

In addition, Mahler's study demonstrated that solutions in the realm of irreality ("magical thinking") have only a small substitute value in real-world task situations. This was also confirmed by the results of a study by Sarah Sliosberg (1934), which tested the substitute value of substitute objects. Playing and real situation are thus functionally clearly separated areas, which usually have no substitute value for each other. Another result of Sliosberg's study was that once a situation has fully developed, it is difficult to accept a substitute, and that it is easier to introduce a substitute as long as the person has not started to deal with the original object.

5.4. Satiation

Satiation is a state in which a person no longer wants to perform a certain activity. It was investigated by Anitra Karsten (1928/1976). Like the other experimenters, she gave the subjects various tasks. The instruction was to "work until you have had enough." In some cases, she forced the subjects to keep working beyond this point. What did she find out?

Satiation does not increase continuously but shows an erratic course. Relative amenity changes with pronounced aversion. With increasing satiation, the subjects tend to introduce variations to the activity. If the subjects then continue a little further with their task, they experience a disintegration of Gestalt, i.e. a disintegration of the situation.

Strong over-satiation leads to restless actions and emotional outbursts. Rejection, and disgust with the activity then remain for a longer time and a co-satiation of neighboring psychic regions is likely.

Satiation is different from fatigue. One can, for example, be energetic again, if the previous activity is incorporated in something new. Activities that have a stronger positive or negative valence are satiated faster than more neutral ones.

***

Thus far, we can summarize as follows:

It is not only needs that are to be considered as psychic driving forces, but also goals and intentions, if a person is sufficiently committed to them. They constitute tension systems that push in the direction of discharge through completion of the task. The more closely an intention or a task is linked to broader and personally significant goals and needs, the stronger and more stable the corresponding tension system proves to be. Since the functioning of the psyche is holistic, the tendency to completion is also effective in the memory. Unfinished tasks therefore increase the person's level of tension and make it more difficult for him or her to turn to other things with full attention and energy.

Whether something appears to be complete or unfinished is not an "objective" matter but is determined by whether it is completed or not in the person's experience. For this, certain conditions can be stated to be relevant, which also means that you can do something specifically to foster a completion. Further, you can see the success of the effort by whether resumption occurs. Life always creates situations in which an action cannot be completed in the original sense. In searching for appropriate substitute solutions, the investigations of Wera Mahler and her colleagues can be helpful. They emphasize the importance of the "degree of reality" and, most importantly, the significance of "social fact" for the effectiveness of a substitute solution.

We adopt these insights also in psychotherapy when we work with clients who have not been able to bring past situations to a satisfactory completion, and we look for ways to bring them to an inner completion in the here and now, e.g., by encouraging them to write down the unspoken in a letter or to express it in a dialogue with the imagined person in our presence.[14]

The saying "practice makes perfect" is not entirely true. When a (quasi-) need is satisfied and the inner goal of the person is reached, the tension tends to decrease and the drive ceases. Uniform repetitions, which no longer allow the performer to experience further development, lead to over-satiation, thereby resulting in deterioration in performance and strongly negative emotional and motivational consequences. However, we can pay attention to the signs of satiation and provide for variations and variety early by embedding the activity in a different or broader context.

6. Structure of the Psyche, Tension, and Equilibrium

So far, we have mainly dealt with the dynamics of a single tension system, with its emergence, its discharge, and satiation. However, the question remains as to how Lewin conceptualizes the functioning of the psyche as a whole and the cooperation that has to be sustained among manifold needs and quasi-needs. We can hardly assume that such tension systems exist side by side in total isolation and that they only successively come into tension.

The single psychic tensions and energies, therefore, belong to systems, which in themselves represent dynamic units and show a higher or lesser degree of isolation. The quasi-needs in particular, which can be traced back to actions, do not represent isolated mental entities, but are mostly embedded in more comprehensive mental structures and are mostly in close communication with other quasi-needs
and needs.

According to Lewin, we can assume an equilibrium tendency for the psychological field: changes – from an idle state to an event or a change in a stationary equilibrium – are due to the fact that the equilibrium is disturbed, and processes are now starting to push in the direction of a new equilibrium. This equilibrium tendency only applies to the system as a whole; partial processes can run in the opposite direction. Equilibrium in Lewin's theory is therefore not a homeostatic state, but a steady state in which conflicting forces at a certain level of pressure and counterpressure hold the balance.

In recent years, Norbert Andersch (2012) pointed out that Lewin's theory of tension systems was often misinterpreted as a relaxation theory. On the contrary, Lewin's main concern was to clarify where the energies for experience and action come from, how they are organized, and how they coordinate to

---

14 On "unfinished business" cf. Lindorfer & Stemberger (2012), on intrusions and flashbacks Sternek (2016), and on "working with the 'empty chair'" Stemberger (2014).

guarantee people's complex life activity. In that sense, his interest in exploring the tension systems was not primarily about how to support their discharge; on the contrary, it was all about finding out what it takes to build up and hold sufficient tension to be able to pursue goals over longer periods of time and in adverse circumstances.

Therefore, we can say that Lewin's concept of the psyche is about how manifold tension systems can be held in parallel (ibid., 31).

7. Theory of Systems in Tension: Conclusions for Therapeutic Practice

Gestalt theoretical psychotherapy relies mainly on Kurt Lewin's dynamic field theory of personality, in which the understanding of the dynamics of human experience and behavior is addressed. Since Lewin has excluded the question of the relationship of the life space to the non-psychological environment, which is highly relevant for psychotherapy and the question of how people can interact at all, his concept is "reinterpreted" by taking critical-realistic assumptions into account. This led to Stemberger's formulation of the multiple-field approach in psychotherapy (2018c).

Psychotherapy aims to help clients alleviate or overcome suffering. It is a collaborative, interactive endeavor of at least one therapist and one client, with the therapeutic relationship playing a central role. Client and therapist enter into a communication and relationship process that is intended to help the client to better understand herself/himself, to build up resources, and to find suitable solutions to her/his problems. The coordination between the interaction partners in the psychotherapeutic process can be understood as a field event ("psychotherapeutic field"). However, unlike, for example, psychoanalytic conceptions that took up Lewin's concept of field (Baranger & Baranger 2008; Ferro 2003; Katz 2017; cf. Stemberger 2019), Gestalt theoretical psychotherapy emphasizes that we have to assume two psychotherapeutic fields: a psychotherapeutic field in the phenomenal world of the client and a psychotherapeutic field in the phenomenal world of the therapist. These can differ significantly from each other. What happens in the therapist's phenomenal world first has to become a fact in the client's phenomenal world in order to have any influence.[15] This fact then can have a completely different function in the psychotherapeutic field of the client as compared to that in the psychotherapeutic field of the therapist (Stemberger 2019, 64). With this in mind, the therapist has to constantly exchange interactions with the client to be able to do his/her job.

---

[15] More details on how the transmission of communication content between the phenomenal worlds of interacting people can be conceptualized in the critical-realistic model can be found in Bischof (1966) and Tholey (1986/2018); cf. also Sternek 2021.

According to the field-theoretical approach, GTP focuses on the psychological situation of the client and not on particular events, symptoms, or personality traits. ●e peculiarities of individual parts or characteristics are considered to be determined by the character of the psychological situation as a whole (Stemberger 2018a). Thus, the field-theoretical approach is not aimed at changing one single aspect, but at changing the overall situation, mainly by recentering or other forms of restructuring of the situation. Through reference to the field-theoretical "principle of contemporaneity" (Lewin, 1936, 34) of the acting forces, we derive the understanding that the focus is on the here-and-now, including the psychological future and the psychological past as they are given therein.

Translated into praxeology, this requires, first, that the client achieves clarity about herself, her/his world, and her/his possibilities for action. The Gestalt-theoretical therapist supports this by "practicing phenomenology" with the client (Stemberger 2016). This means to help the client to explore her/his phenomenal world by seeing, hearing, feeling, sensing in an open, receptive attitude and taking the perceived, the felt, and the sensed seriously. The task of the therapist is to stimulate, support, and guide the client in this process. Because there is no direct access to the world of others, client and therapist are constantly reliant on exchange and dialog in this process.

If "practicing phenomenology" is about exploring "what is" and therefore addresses the phenomenal world of the client, the so-called "force field analysis" addresses the forces acting on the life space. These forces cannot be perceived directly, but only through their effects. One could say that in this step, we are supporting the client to explore "what operates" in her/his world: What are the needs, goals, wishes, and intentions that underlie the forces? Do these needs, goals, and wishes have their origin in the client or are they induced from "others," who might be parents, partners, superiors, or society? What effects do they have on her/his experience and behavior, and how do they relate to the client's possibilities and situational requirements? The "field force analysis" in GTP is, of course, not a scientific but an experience-oriented analysis. Therefore, it is more an experimental than an intellectual undertaking. It takes advantage of the fact that with exploration and experimentation, the balance of forces in the field is already changing. This is one reason why in GTP we speak of the method of "change-activating" force-field analysis. The therapist develops his/her suggestions for experiments depending on the circumstances and requirements of the specific situation and thereby focuses on the relationships outside of therapy or the client–therapist relationship, as appropriate (cf. Böhm 2021, 2022). However, the findings and results of the studies of the Lewin group can serve him/her as an orientation- and idea-generator.

Lewin's theory of tension systems has sharpened our focus, especially on the positive, constructive side of tension in people's lives. Thus, they counterbalance the one-sided overemphasis of relaxation in many psychological approaches. Living systems need tension to be able to exist at all – without tension they are no longer alive. In terms of psychotherapy, the task in many cases is not only to help bring about relaxation and the release of energy for something new through completion of unfinished projects, but to do much more to support clients in building up and sustaining tensions, which they need in order to pursue important life tasks (Lindorfer & Stemberger 2012). As we learned from the experimental work of the Lewin group, in this context, sufficient stability, a connection of goals with ego-near needs, and the ability to engage are significant.

Finally, where unfinished business burdens clients, the results of the experimental research give us clues as to how we can provide a conclusion: similarity to the inner goal, the greatest possible degree of reality (in the form of action or the creation of social facts), and an adequate degree of difficulty. The latter also relates to the case where someone sets his goals too high in relation to his inner and outer possibilities.

4. Ego and Self in Gestalt Theory

Gerhard Stemberger[16]

Summary

The paper presents basic Gestalt theoretical concepts of ego and self. They differ from other concepts in that they do not comprehend ego and self as fixed entities or as central controlling instances of the psyche, but as one specific organized unit in a psychological field in dynamic interrelation with the other organized units - the environment units - of this field. On this theme, well-known representatives of Gestalt theory have presented some general and special theories since the early days of this approach that could partly be substantiated experimentally. They illuminate the relationship between ego and world in everyday life as well as in the case of mental disorders. Not only the spatial extension of the phenomenal ego is subject to situational changes, but also its place in the world, its functional fitting in this world, its internal differentiation, its permeability to the environment and much more. The German Gestalt psychologist Wolfgang Metzger emphasizes the significant functional role that this dynamic plasticity of the phenomenal world and its continuously changing segregation of ego and environment have for human life by designating the phenomenal world as a "Central Steering Mechanism". In this article, ego and self as part of this field in their interrelation with the total psychological field will be illuminated from the perspective of the thinking of the Gestalt psychologists Max Wertheimer, Kurt Koffka, Wolfgang Köhler, Kurt Lewin, Wolfgang Metzger, Mary Henle, Edwin Rausch and Giuseppe Galli.

"The genesis of an Ego ..."

"... the genesis of an Ego is one of the strangest and most remarkable of phenomena which, it would appear, is also controlled by whole-processes", Max Wertheimer, the founder of Gestalt theory, once observed (Wertheimer 1924 in 1944, 90).

And indeed, hardly anyone ponders in daily life or pays attention to in other ways, whether or not there might be such a thing as an ego. In our lives it is just there either a matter of course, or as an implicit point of reference for the spatial coordinates "in front of me", "next to me", "behind me" - or sometimes it is not there at all.

There are situations in which the ego is "everything" - where about in the raging pain, hardly another world exists besides the ego. There are situations where the ego spatially expands and subsumes otherwise separated areas of the environment, such as the clothing, the car, sporting equipment, and again other

---

[16] The article – first published 2021 in the journal *Gestalt Theory*, 41(1), 46-67 – is loosely based on the lecture "The Phenomenal Ego and its World" at the Symposium "100 Years of Gestalt Psychology" in Helsinki, 28.-29.9.2012. I thank Ed Ragsdale, Ian Verstegen, and Michael Wertheimer for reviewing earlier drafts and for encouraging its publication. The remaining deficiencies remain my responsibility.

situations in which it involuntarily or voluntarily dwindles away, possibly shrinks to a small point, or in extreme cases, becomes disembodied. At times the ego is the center of its world, then again marginal, sometimes it functions as a member of a larger whole, such as in a team sport or in a well-coordinated working group, then again there are situations where another person serves as an "extension" of one's will, or even as an extension of one's ego.[17]

Everyday experience already shows that the ego is not a solid, more or less steady "object", but something very mutable in many ways. Our life would obviously not be possible at all without this high plasticity and constant changeability of the ego in a flow of constantly changing situations and their demands.

Our ego may be experienced, or it may be functionally present without being experienced. It may take center stage or may take a very marginal place in our phenomenal world. It may also assume quite different functional roles in the phenomenal world – perhaps subordinated as part of a larger whole, acting as a specific limb for some complex activity, or in the role of a subordinate element in a collective action, or fully identified with a purpose itself, or even dissolve in the demands of a specific situation. It may vary in its permeability with respect to its phenomenal world. It may vary in the extent and strength of the internal differentiation of its inner "regions" or "layers", which may also vary in their level of interaction with each other and with the phenomenal environment: It consists of manifold dynamic internal and external interactions and thus finely regulates its internal life, and likewise its relations with the phenomenal environment, especially also with the fellow human beings. Its energy level and state of tension will vary in accord with its specific objectives. Under certain conditions the ego may double or multiply, with each of these phenomenal egos having its own phenomenal environment - just think of "daydreaming" or a visit to the cinema, in which you may be "drawn" into the thrilling movie action with the result that you (your first ego) can sit in your seat in the auditorium (the environment of your first ego)

---

[17] The whole variety of relevant Gestalt psychological research in this area unfortunately cannot be presented here for reasons of space. Some of it should be referred to at least briefly. The work of the German Gestalt psychologists Kurt Kohl (1956) and Paul Tholey (1989, 1990, 2018) in sports psychology deserves mention. They investigated the "coalescence" of the athlete with the sports equipment (or even with the relevant environment, such as the ski slope) and to the inclusion of the self in a structured We in team sports. Furthermore, the lucid dream research of Paul Tholey (2018) and others have contributed extensively to a differentiated understanding of the phenomenal self. The work of the German Gestalt psychologist Edwin Rausch on the perception of paintings (Rausch 1982) gave the impetus to the development of the multiple-field approach in Gestalt Theoretical Psychotherapy (cf. Stemberger 2009, 2018c, 2022b).

on the one hand as the moviegoer, and on the other hand you (your second ego) simultaneously live and act as the adventurer in a completely different world (the environment of the second ego).

Any changes in that area of the phenomenal field that forms our phenomenal ego, inevitably results in corresponding changes in the field of its phenomenal environment - and vice versa - in an unceasing dynamic interrelationship. If the ego is central, its environment would be peripheral - and vice versa. If it expands, its phenomenal environment would shrink - and vice versa. The tensions of its needs and intentions lead to specific changes in its experienced environment, and vice versa the occurrence of corresponding issues in his experienced environment provides opportunities and impetus for relaxation or "transformation" of its needs. Changes of its world can originate, at times, due to the ego's activity, or at other times, without its active involvement. And in all of this, the phenomenal processes are intimately intertwined via action and "feedback" with the physiological organism and its physical environment, including the other people and organisms in it.

Early Gestalt Psychology Contributions

The dynamic variability of the phenomenal ego and its phenomenal environment, as well as the terms of their relative phenomenal constancy and the way they interact with the rest of the physical world, have been subjects of discussion in Gestalt theory dating from the early work of its founders.[18] I would like to refer to three of these early contributions first - already these show that Gestalt theory was from the very beginning an approach that anticipated all the important moments of today's debate in cognitive science about embodied, embedded, extended, and enactive cognition (the "4E cognition") with original approaches that deserve more attention.

As a first reference for this I mention the explanation of the genesis and cure of a case of paranoid disorder, given by the German psychiatrist Heinrich Schulte inspired by Max Wertheimer[19] (Schulte 1924 in 1986): In this case an ego, experiencing itself as completely segregated from the others and suffering from this situation in an intolerable manner, manages to get into the very

---

[18] Some of the terminological and conceptual differences in the consideration of ego and self among the founders of Gestalt psychology, not covered in this paper, are discussed by A.S. Luchins 1961.

[19] Wertheimer's assistant and collaborator Erwin Levy: „The author in fact was Max Wertheimer, who years later told me that he had outlined the theory to Dr. Schulte, who was to work it out in final form." Levy 1986, 230. We therefore speak of the „Schulte/Wertheimer theses".

center of the situation and into a strong relationship with the group through a radical paranoid restructuring of the situation as this ego perceives it.

As a second reference, I will address the Berlin experimental program of "Investigations in the Psychology of Action and Emotion" (1926–1937) of Kurt Lewin and his students: Here the mental tension systems and the structure and dynamics of the ego-environment division are at the center of diverse experiments on laws governing human behavior.[20]

For a third example, we will take a closer look at Kurt Koffka's Gestalt theory of the ego, the first and most systematic early treatment of the subject from a Gestalt theoretical perspective (in Koffka's "Principles" 1935).

Disturbances in the Ego-World Relationship

Sometimes, unexpected disturbances of usual processes and situations reveal their otherwise unnoticed dynamic order and functioning in ordinary life. Therefore (and also because in my field, psychotherapy, we are mostly confronted with disturbances and their painful consequences) let me start with some examples of such disturbances in the relationship of the ego and its world. As the following examples show, the disturbance can take its origin from a functionally inappropriate positioning of the ego in its world, or from an inappropriate fusion of the ego with parts of its world, or from an either too high or too low reciprocal permeability of the environment regions and the ego-regions, or the disorder may manifest itself in a problematic interrelation between simultaneously existing multiple phenomenal worlds. These four cases probably contain the most important constellations according to clinical experience, nevertheless there is no reason to regard the list as conclusive.

Let me now give you four examples of how these constellations can practically manifest themselves in certain life difficulties and mental disorders:

1. Problems arising from inappropriate positioning of the ego in its world:

As already mentioned, the paranoid delusions are understood by Schulte/Wertheimer as a disturbed Ego-We-organization. In this case (Schulte 1924 in 1986). a tatar war prisoner in WW I finds himself in an unbearable marginal position excluded from the We of the other war prisoners because nobody understands his language and he does not understand the others. As a prisoner, he cannot escape from this unbearable situation. A process of restructuring the situation – as he experiences it – sets in for him. The tatar prisoner finally

---

[20] For an overview see Lewin's "Survey of Experimental Investigations", Lewin 1935, 239–273; the translation and discussion of some of these studies can be found in De Rivera 1976; for a discussion of further continuation of this approach, see Lindorfer 2021.

perceives himself in the very center of the situation as being the person perse-cuted by all the others. This is by no means a comfortable solution for him but one which is more bearable than being completely cut off from the others in a situation which demands so strongly a We-affiliation of some kind. This mental restructuring of the situation comprises not only a change of locus of the ego in its phenomenal world, but also a total reorganization of all the functional rela-tions in the environmental field.

2. Problems arising from a boundary violating, in extreme cases even abusive behavior of a person,

who perceives other people as an extension of its own ego: Such a person has "incorporated" the other, made him a part of its own ego, or uses the other as a "continuation" or "extension" of its own ego, as for example a mere tool. Here an expansion of the ego, incorporating other persons, combines with a correspond-ing functional rearrangement of the complete phenomenal field, which is per-ceived as being structured entirely in the service of its own immediate interests. Such inclusion of the other in one's own person need not be linked to a negative, abusive context, but is in other situations a completely normal, functionally de-manded and useful process. Koffka mentioned, for example, the initial inclusion of the infant in the ego of the mother, as indicated by her tendency to react the same way regardless of whether she herself or her child is placed in a particular situation. This initially is a perfectly sensible and functional structural character-istic of the field, however, it may become problematic and conflictual to the ex-tent that the mother's incorporation of her child as part of herself comes to clash with the child's own growing independence. Similar constellations can be ob-served in intimate personal relationships of adults, but also in all other areas of working, social, and political life, in both positive and negative manifestations.

3. Disturbances of the functional relationship between parts of the phenome-nal field:

Stuttering is usually associated with a specific disorder of the whole-relation-ship in the phenomenal world: fluency of speech requires that the attention is focused on the other and on the relationship to this other and not on the tech-nical process of speaking or even on the organs of speech. Again, we are deal-ing here with a restructuring of the phenomenal world, in which the function-ally meaningful relationships between the parts and the whole in the field are disturbed.

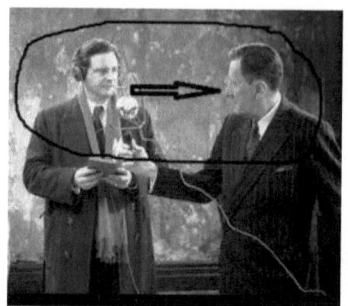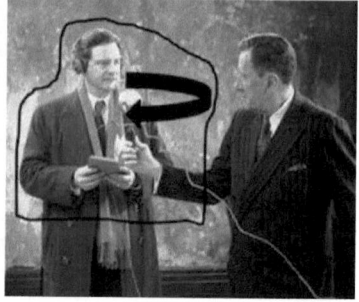

Fig: The situation of stuttering: fluent speech requires that the focus of attention is on the other person and the relationship to him (Fig. 1) and not on the speech process or even on the speech organs (Fig. 2). (GSt after a screenshot from the movie "The King's Speech")

4. Disturbances in the relationship of multiple total fields:

The research of Gestalt psychologist Edwin Rausch has shown (Rausch 1982), that under certain conditions the ego-environment-structure of the phenomenal field differentiates further and a second phenomenal ego segregates with a second phenomenal world, for instance in "daydreaming", mental sports training, "mind wandering" and similar processes (Stemberger 2009, 2018c, 2022b). The interrelationship between these two total fields can have a constructive effect (for example for problem solving) but can also be part of a problematic process. Eating disorders, for example, are understood by Thomas Fuchs as solidifying the segregation of a second phenomenal total field with a second phenomenal ego to maintain a liveable balance in an otherwise difficult or even unbearable situation (see Fuchs 2010, 2021).

The basic position of critical realism

The Gestalt theoretical conception of a close correlation between an ever-adapting and therefore (within certain limits) changing phenomenal world and an equally – within certain limits – variable ego, is closely related to the epistemological core position of Gestalt theory, critical realism:

According to this basic position, first formulated by Köhler 1929 (see Figure 3), it is necessary to clearly distinguish between, on the one hand, a) the phenomenal world, encountered in experience (with a phenomenal bodily ego segregated within this phenomenal world), and on the other hand, b) the transphenomenal world, including the physiological organism within his physical environment.[21]

---

[21] In Koffka's terminology this is the differentiation of "geographical world" and "behavioural world". (Koffka 1935, 40 ff) Cf. Sternek in this volume for a more detailed account of critical realism.

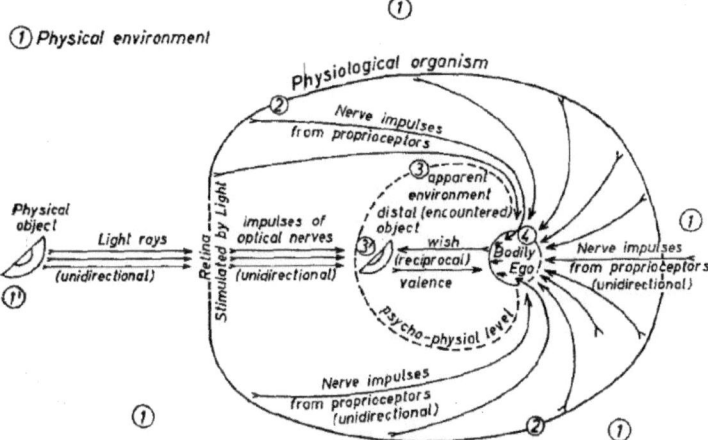

Figure 3: Schema of ego-environment relations (after Köhler 1929), in the graphic representation of Metzger 2001, 283, in English in Metzger 1972, 244. Relationship between physical world including physiological organism (= Macrocosm) and phenomenal-perceptual world including experienced bodily Ego (= Microcosm)

1 = physical environment of organism; 1' = physical object, reflecting light rays; 2 = physiological organism, as part of the physical world; 3 = apparent (perceived) environment of bodily Ego; 3' = = apparent (distal) object or percept, representing the physical object; 4 = bodily Ego, as part of the phenomenal-perceptual world, representing the organism

The physiological organism and its physical environment provide via nervous and brain processes the material basis for the phenomenal world of each person. Between both worlds, the transphenomenal and the phenomenal, constant coordination processes take place that are needed for life and survival of the human being in its physical environment. The person can experience some of the workings and effects of this transphenomenal side of his existence in his phenomenal world but has no immediate experiential access to it.

The phenomenal world of each person is a microcosm within the macrocosm of the physical world. These microcosms are part of the physical macrocosm but have specific features – phenomenal and dynamic qualities – other parts of the physical world do not have. Gestalt theory holds that the phenomenal world is in fact not just a more or less good and veridical "image" of the physical world but has the dynamic characteristics of a field. This field is mainly organized by the needs and quasi-needs of the phenomenal ego on the one hand, the attractive and repulsive qualities in its phenomenal environment on the other. The facts appearing and occurring in the phenomenal world stand not unrelated to each other, but in close dynamic (field-like) interaction with each other. They are not neutral but are experienced as attractive or repulsive and organize according to the given total field situation and the constant cybernetic interaction of the phenomenal world with the organism and its physical environment, their constant influences and feedback. It is this peculiarity which makes the phenomenal world apt to function as the "central steering mechanism" of the human organism in its physical environment and along the same path to interaction with other humans which interact in the same way from their microcosms with the common physical environment.

A model of "super-veridical representation"

At this point, a brief side glance at the debate in the cognitive sciences is allowed, whether representationalist models or non-representationalist models do better justice to the human cognitive process. In my opinion, such confrontations have not proved fruitful (cf. Verstegen 2012). With its critical realist model Gestalt theory offers an alternative. It assumes that man with his phenomenal world has at his disposal an embodied microcosm which not only represents veridically to an astonishingly high degree the part of the macrocosm surrounding him which is relevant for him in his given life situation but can do much more. It can not only represent its macro-physical environment like a veridical picture or film recording, it can do beyond that what no film camera of the world can do: It can create a representation of this world in constant flux, in which not only this world, but simultaneously also his own relationship to this world and the dynamic development of this relationship is represented in constant interaction. In this sense the microcosm of man is not only veridical, it is *super-veridical,* insofar as it is able to represent veridically not only the objects surrounding man and the influence of his actions on these objects, but beyond that also his personal dynamic relation to these objects ((including the most significant "objects" for him, his fellow people). Only this super-veridicality enables this microcosm to serve as a steering organ for man's experience and behavior in the macrocosm, which surrounds him and of which he is an active part.

The "Central Steering Mechanism"

I adopt here the term "Central Steering Mechanism" from Wolfgang Metzger.[22] In 1969 he asked the question:

---

[22] Lewin 1935 has already pointed out the steering role of the perceptual field, referring to Köhler 1922 and Lewin & Sakuma 1925: "Thus there occurs a *steering* of the process by the perceptual field." (Lewin 1935, 48) Metzger, however, deserves credit for having elaborated this idea conceptually in a systematic way.

"What is the use of this duplication of the world into a physical and a perceptive one, of the person into an organism and a bodily ego, of stimulation into configurations of physico-chemical impacts upon receptors and valences affecting the ego, and of reaction into intended changes of the bodily ego and motions executed by parts of the organism? What relevance can all this have? It is extremely improbable that so highly complicated an organization could have developed during evolution and preserved without a considerable survival value." (Metzger 1972, 247).

Metzger answered that question as follows:

"The function of the phenomenal world, then, would be to make possible just those dynamic interactions and to transfer them to the organism through an intricate system of circular conductors that allow for the necessary feedback in such a way that the organism itself is made to behave 'with regard to' the objects encountered in its environment and relevant for its survival." (ibid, 249)

To explain this, Metzger chooses as an example a goal-directed body movement. If a person wants to reach for a water glass, the movement of his phenomenal hand towards the phenomenal water glass leads to the corresponding movement of his respective physiological limb towards the physical object "water glass". Appropriate cybernetic feedback processes control the physiological movement and the continuous feedback about the successful coordination between the movement of the phenomenal hand and the movement of the physiological hand.

"My intention to lift up my right hand, e.g., can only be directed to the phenomenal hand as a part of my phenomenal bodily ego but never directly to the anatomical part of my organism that is related to the former and bears the same name." (ibid, 245) That there are significant differences between the experienced arm and the corresponding physiological part of the organism, becomes somewhat obvious from the "discrepancy between the region of the bodily ego on which our will immediately acts, and the region of the organism that, at the same time, is subject to innervation. [...] the former region lies unmistakeably within the hand itself as a part of the bodily ego, whereas the latter just as unmistakeably lies within the muscular system of the upper arm and the shoulder of the anatomical organism." (ibid, 245)

"The interrelations between the subject and the object, [...] become themselves a steering mechanism, in which—in the case of attraction—the place of the phenomenal object represents the value aimed at, the position of the subject the actual value, and consequently the distance between them represents the difference between these two values by which the human steering machine viz. the muscular system is set in motion so that in the physical world the distance between the organism and the object diminishes and finally disappears.." (ibid, 251)

Metzger points out the similarity of this steering function to a servomechanism, for example the mechanical steering of a large vessel, emphasizes, however, that this similarity is limited.

This steering process depends, of course, on whether and how the central nervous and peripheral nervous connections required for it between the corresponding phenomenal processes and the organism are active. This is largely not the case during sleep, for example, where as a consequence movements of the dream body do not lead to corresponding movements of the organism. To a large extent this kind of connection is also shut down for those areas of the phenomenal world, which have segregated as a second total field of experience with its own phenomenal ego, for example during a "daydream". Metzger mentions also other examples where it does not come to such a coupling of phenomenal motions and motions of the physiological organism: "in the hallucinations of motion due to affections of the brain by psychoses, lesions, or poisoning, as well as in the illusory movement of phantom-limbs after amputation." (ibid, 245)

Of course, Metzger's example of an arm movement is just a very simple example of how the phenomenal world of man acts as a central steering system. Not only bodily movements, but the whole manoeuvring of man in his environment, from the simplest life and species-sustaining activities such as food procurement, securing his physical integrity, reproduction, etc., up to the most complex interactions in his interpersonal environment would according to this thesis be controlled by this kind of interaction between the phenomenal world, its organism and its other physical environment.

Mind you: This steering function is attributed by Metzger to the phenomenal world in its entirety - not primarily, or even solely to the phenomenal self within this phenomenal world. In this point, Gestalt theory differs significantly from many other approaches that deal with the ego and attribute to the ego a much "more prominent" role, as does Gestalt theory. To characterize these Gestalt theoretical positions, I will sketch now some key ideas of relevant representatives.

Max Wertheimer: "strange and most remarkable"

As early as 1924 in his famous lecture "Gestalt theory" before the Kant society Max Wertheimer made the following remark – which might sound a bit strange for contemporary ears:

"Here I am – the Ego – first a part of the field. I am not fundamentally an Ego standing in relief against other Egos, as has usually been maintained; no, the genesis of an Ego is one of the strangest and most remarkable of phenomena which, it would appear, is also controlled by whole-processes. As I have stated, I am a part in this field." (Wertheimer 1924 in 1944, 90)

Here, in this early presentation of Gestalt theory, Wertheimer already postulates some basic theses, which are characteristic for the Gestalt theoretical conception of the ego (later on elaborated in more detail, especially by Koffka):

First: An ego neither exists from the outset in the experience and behavior of humans nor does it exist always, but it is formed only under certain conditions. This remark does not, or at least not primarily, refer to the developmental process of the genesis of an ego-experience in infancy (cf. for this topic Arfelli Galli 2012). Rather, it states also for the adult that an "I versus the others" is experienced only under certain conditions. His ego may, for example, under certain conditions, at least for some time dissolve entirely in a group, or forget about himself completely in a specific activity.

And secondly: This ego does not unfold as a psychic apparatus, "command center" or the like, e.g. an agency that does and controls everything. Instead, this ego forms as a field-part - as part of the psychological field of experience and behavior - and abides by the same "laws of the whole" (i.e. Gestalt factors) as all the rest of the experiential and behavioral world.

This conception of the self in Gestalt theory viewing the ego as a field part besides and interrelated with other field parts appears quite unpretentious compared with much weightier conceptions of the ego as a powerful psychic apparatus and the like. This has prompted the Italian Gestalt psychologist Giuseppe Galli in later years to speak of a "narcissistic deflation" of this concept in Gestalt theory as opposed to the "narcissistic inflation of the ego" in other theories (Galli 2005, 46).

But Wertheimer goes even further:

"Man is not only part of a field, but a part and member of his group. When people are together, as when they are at work, then the most unnatural behavior, which only appears in late stages or abnormal cases, would be to behave as separate Egos. Under normal circumstances they work in common, each a meaningfully functioning part of the whole. Consider South Sea Islanders working together, or children at play. An Ego standing vis a vis or in contrast to the others usually develops only under very special circumstances." (Wertheimer 1924 in 1944, 92)

Wertheimer links this to the assumption:

"If for any outward or inner reasons a harmonious balance is not attainable between a person and the people with whom he lives, then definite disturbances of the equilibrium must appear and in extreme instances lead to precarious substitutes for the natural equilibrium which will transform the psychological structure of that person. This led to the hypothesis that a wide range of mental disease, for which no actual theory had previously been submitted, might be the consequence of such fundamental processes." (ibid)

This hypothesis has been elaborated in depth in the aforementioned treatise of the German psychiatrist Heinrich Schulte, under supervision of Max Wertheimer, on the origin and cure of a case of paranoid disorder (see Schulte 1924 in 1986).

Thirdly, therefore: As far as the phenomenal ego in its phenomenal world is concerned, there are special relations of belonging and centering with regard to its fellow human beings. These fellow men are of particular importance for man in comparison to other issues and facts in his world; therefore humans (or shapes that resemble people) are particularly highlighted in everyday perception (even in the case where there are no humans: just think of the "man on the moon") – man needs his fellowmen most essentially for his life and survival. These relations of belonging and centering in his phenomenal world are therefore in most cases the decisive factor for loosing and for regaining mental health.

Kurt Koffka on ego and self

Therefore, from the Gestalt theoretical point of view, the phenomenal ego is a field-part that is segregated from the phenomenal field. This field-part is more or less closely interrelated to all other parts of the field, as well as the field as a whole. Kurt Koffka systematically explained this concept in 1935 in his major work *"Principles of Gestalt Psychology"* (especially in chapter 8) and further elaborated on it.

In a letter to his long-time collaborator Molly Harrower on March 24th, 1933, Koffka already characterizes his ego-concept in four key statements:

"**One**: The phenomenal Ego and the phenomenal environment are a segregated field part.

Two: When Ego disappears from the phenomenal world or consciousness ceases altogether, the need tensions within the Ego system survive.

Three: Therefore, the real, psycho-physical Ego is not identical with the phenomenal Ego, but it is permanent. This persistance of the Ego is not memory in the usual sense, but comparable to the persistence of the real organism in the real environment. This makes a theory of personality possible.

Four: If the Ego as a segregated system persists independently of consciousness, then the environment from which it is segregated must also persist independently of consciousness. Otherwise, there would be nothing to segregate and unify the Ego system ". (Harrower 1983, 31f)

According to Koffka (on this point heavily relying on Kurt Lewin) the phenomenal ego is made up of tension systems, which are in constant interaction with the environment. These tension systems owe their existence to the needs and quasi-needs (a term Lewin uses for the conscious and non-conscious intentions) of people. Depending on the possibilities of satisfying these needs and quasi-needs or of finding some substitute satisfaction – these possibilities depending on what the environment has to offer but also on the personality structure and dynamics - the processes originating from these tension systems will eventually result in a relaxation of the subsystems in play, leading to a redistribution of tension in the entire system (see Lindorfer & Stemberger 2012, Lindorfer 2021, also in this volume).

Thus, this constant process of satisfaction, partial satisfaction, substitute-satisfaction or non-satisfaction of needs and quasi needs is accompanied by a constant change in the tension systems that make up the ego in its relationship with its environment. In this interaction, there must necessarily be constant changes of the field part ego just as changes of the surrounding field parts.

But there is not only variability in these processes; there is also a certain constancy of structural and dynamic characteristics which is reflected in the experience of identity of oneself and of the world over time. Therefore, as far as the ego is concerned, we are dealing according to Koffka on one hand with various temporary sub-systems of the ego, on the other with a relatively enduring subsystem of the ego, a core-ego, which is now referred to as the "Self" by Koffka:

"The sub-systems do not simply exist side by side; they are organized in various ways. One principle of organization is that of surface-depth organization. The Ego has a core, the Self, and enveloping this core, in various communications with it and each other, are other sub-systems, comparable to different layers, until we come to the surface, which is most easily touched, and most easily discharged. Another principle of organization concerns the communication between the different systems, a third relative dominance." (Koffka 1935, 342)

Koffka on the internal structure of the ego

Koffka discusses in detail the question as to what conditions determine the segregation of a phenomenal ego as a separate field-part within the phenomenal total field. He presents the case of an Austrian mountaineer who fell in a crevasse, losing consciousness, then only gradually awakening from unconsciousness. This mountaineer described afterwards how in this process there was first no ego at all and how then an ego came into existence. From the description of this process Koffka concludes that the body perceptions of primarily proprioceptive nature seem to have played a decisive role in this case for the segregation of a phenomenal ego from the rest of the phenomenal field. These body perceptions brought sufficient non-homogeneity into the originally homogeneous field. Following certain Gestalt principles (especially the factors of proximity, similarity, and common fate), these body perceptions enabled the fusion of a region of the field as sufficiently different from the rest of the field. Thus, they brought about the collapse of the first unified field in a bi-polar field, having the two poles ego and non-ego. One pole – forming the "core of the self" – attracts all the bodily experiences and gives rise to the emergence of a bodily ego while the auditory and visual experiences remain on the "external pole" and thus belong to the environment part of the field.

"How this point-core itself was formed, we do not know. It must have had a great deal to do with the victim's earlier Ego [Koffka is talking about the mountain climber fallen in the crevasse], his wishes, fears, determinations, which are now brought into play. " (Koffka 1935, 324f)

In 1936 Koffka writes to Harrower again on this topic:

„What factors are responsible for Ego organization? What kind of properties must processes have in order to operate in the Ego? From this point of view the normal and pathological case is equally in need of explanation. ... We do not necessarily have to search for Intra Ego forces but may envisage the whole structure of the person's mind, including both Ego and Environment processes, and looking for special characteristics in either field. " (Harrower 1983, 127f)

This shows that Koffka considers it important to deal also with the internal structure of the ego whose core he addresses as the self. This subsystem "self" is characterized according to Koffka by much stronger stresses than the other (temporary) subsystems of the ego: He thinks that the reason for this is that these stresses correspond to real needs, as opposed to the tensions of quasi-needs which arise from more superficial and temporary intentions (Koffka 1935, 342).

As an example of the dynamic importance of the internal structure of the ego, Koffka refers to the Berlin experiments of Kurt Lewin and his students, especially to the work of Bluma Zeigarnik (1927):

"For an ambitious person to miss the solution of a problem means 'failure', means that the achievement has fallen below his 'personal standard', means therefore a definite affection of that part of the Ego system which we shall now call the 'self'." (Koffka 1935, 341).

Köhler: Small objection, big approval

Wolfgang Köhler's views differ only slightly from those of Koffka. Only in one point does he announce objection (see Luchins 1961, 21): While Koffka normally situates the thoughts of the person in the ego (1935, 327–329), Köhler cautions against regarding thoughts or thoughts objects as part of the phenomenal ego – this would result in leaving strictly phenomenological grounds and would invite "a most unfortunate vagueness in the use of the term self (Köhler 1938, 90; see there also footnote 2 on Koffka).

Except for this difference Köhler shares the arguments put forward in Koffka's ego-theory in all of its main points. Koffka reports in a further letter to Harrower on 06/15/1933 that he had many good talks with Köhler, and „he agrees with my Ego Theory completely. It did not even seem to be new to him. He finds it as necessary a conclusion as I did, which gave me great satisfaction." (Harrower 1983, 11)

Köhler also shared Koffka's beliefs that the phenomenal ego and its phenomenal environment correspond to a neural ego and a neural environment in the brain processes, and that these in turn account for even just part of the whole brain activity. This aspect is related to the important question, of how to explain how something apparently from my phenomenal ego and also something from my phenomenal environment seems to have a continuing existence even when my self-awareness and my world-awareness are interrupted (in sleep or in unconsciousness) – after waking my phenomenal ego and my phenomenal environment are available again, as if there had not been any interruption of my awareness. This conception of a neural correlate of the phenomenal ego and a neural correlate of its phenomenal environment Köhler himself addresses in 1938 as follows:

"Although many sources contribute to its make-up, the 'subjective' part of the phenomenal field, including the emotional life, the kinaesthetic and the visual components of the self, represents under normal conditions a unit which as such has commerce with the 'objective' world. We are thus forced to postulate a similarly intimate organization and centralization of all the neural events which underlie the phenomenal self. And as the phenomenal self generally represents one entity in its commerce with the 'objective' world, so its complex neural correlate will behave as a unit in its functional relations with the correlates of 'objective' percepts." (Köhler 1938, 354)

Lewin on the internal structure of the ego

Similar to Koffka, Lewin goes after the issue of internal differentiation or internal structure of the ego, as well as its role in relation to the environment. However, Lewin uses a slightly different terminology than Koffka. Where Koffka speaks of the "self," Lewin speaks of an "inner core of personality," of "inner regions of the soul" and "intra-psychic systems," of "deep layers" and terms alike. So Lewin and his students take a topological perspective, the viewpoint of the spatial internal structure of the person. As we have seen, we find this perspective also in Koffka's writings where he speaks of surface and depth, layers and core etc.

Lewin represents in any case the

"view that a special region, within the psychical totality, must be defined as the self in the narrower sense. Not every psychically existent system would belong to this central self. Not every one to whom I say 'Du,' not all the things, men, and environmental regions which I know and which may perhaps be very important to me, belong to my self. This self-system would also have in functional respects – this is most important – a certain unique position. Not every tense psychical system would stand in communication with this self. Tensions which have to do with the self would also have functionally a special significance in the total psychical organism (…), and it is possible that within this region differently directed tensions would tend to equilibrium considerably more strongly and that relatively isolated dynamic systems within it could much less readily occur." (Lewin 1935, 61f)

In this context Lewin and his students speak of "intra-psychic districts" or "intrapsychic systems" (Dembo 1931 in 1976, 405), further of an "inner core of personality" ("Ich-Kern") within the "deeper layers" of the person (Dembo 1931 in 1976 109; see there also Figure 17).

These more central layers of the ego-core are usually "functionally enclosed". In certain situations, however, with increasing affectivity stresses can break though to these deeper layers of the person (see Dembo 1931 in 1976, 407).

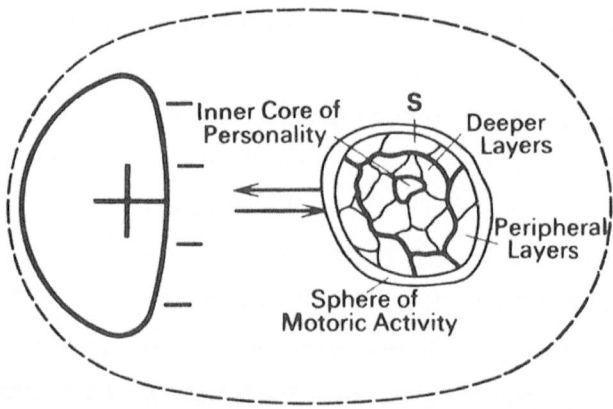

Figure 17 from Dembo 1931 in 1976, *The Dynamics of Anger*, 406

Ferdinand Hoppe, another student of Lewin, further elaborates on the dynamic importance of the internal structure of the ego, describing the dynamic relationship of the ego-core (the "central I") and the levels of aspiration (Hoppe

1930 in 1976, 482f). In this context, Hoppe forms the concept of "ego levels" for the self-worth (ibid, 481, 483–485). According to him, there is a dynamic relationship between the level of aspiration for the particular task at hand and an ego-level, which goes beyond the single task and on which one's own person as a social being is based (ibid, 483; see also the dynamics of the ego-level, the trend to keep it as high as possible, 484).

Mary Henle: the self as a system of related functions

The American Gestalt psychologist Mary Henle, the most important collaborator of Wolfgang Köhler in the USA, draws attention to a further important aspect. She sees in the self a system of closely related functions:

"The most obvious fact about the self as we experience it is the multiplicity of aspects it presents. We do not ordinarily appear to ourselves as an undifferentiated "I"." (Henle 1962, 396). And: "It seems that even when we confine ourselves to what is phenomenally present, the self consists of a variety of functions. [...] Although we often tend to personify them, actually they are functions, not entities." (ibid, 397)

Of such functions Henle gives the following examples: observing and acting, criticizing, accepting or rejecting, [the inner friend: comforting, encouraging], Protecting / adorning / embellishing, realistically assessing / imagining, dreaming ... (see for more details Henle 1962).

On the relationship between the various aspects of self Henle says: "... although conflicts are experiences, as in some of the examples given above, these experientially distinct aspects of the self work together, on the whole, in an organized manner, with reference to each other if not always in harmony." (Henle 1962, 400)

Here one can see a bridge connecting Henle's and Koffka's thinking: Koffka had found that the body perceptions of a primarily proprioceptive nature play a decisive role for the segregation of the phenomenal bodily ego from the rest of the phenomenal field. In line with this, one can proceed, including Henle's reflections on the functions of the self:

For his orientation and ability to act in the world, in particular in his co-human environment, man does not need only "outward directed sense organs" and "intra-corporeal senses", but also functions like a permanent self-reflection, self-examination and self-care, directed towards his phenomenal ego in its identity and in its relationship with its environment. These functions in the ego-region of the field are of paramount importance for the "fine-tuning" of the phenomenal world as a "central steering organ" (Metzger), especially for all human interactions in life. Henle gives some examples which point in this direction in her references to the correlation between self-criticism and response to "external" criticism or on the relationship between self-acceptance (being one's own "inner friend") and having "outer" friends.

Edwin Rausch: Multiple egos – multiple fields

At least briefly, reference must be made here to Edwin Rausch's research on the multiplicity of the ego in perception. Henle's findings have a complement in the function of the multi-field division of the phenomenal world, as we find it in a considerably large part of the waking life of man. As Edwin Rausch has found out in his experimental research (Rausch 1982), it comes to the formation of a second ego with its own phenomenal environment, if in one's primary world of experience circumstances occur, which are not compatible in one and the same world (an effect of the Prägnanz tendency). This is subsequently connected with a sometimes closer, sometimes looser interdependence and interaction between these two total fields and thus also between the two phenomenal egos. The relations between the ego in the primary total field and the ego in the secondary total field can show many of Henle's functions of the ego "in action". For example, the ego in the secondary total field of a wish-fulfilling daydream or in co-experiencing with the hero in a film or novel may be the ego that the ego in the primary total field could not stand up to its own criticism. Or it may be already the decisive condition for the segregation of the second total field that one discovers the experience of another own ego, which cannot be reconciled in one and the same world – at least not immediately and only the interaction between the two egos in the primary and secondary total field makes their later unification possible.

I can only hint at these connections here and refer to the more extensive Gestalt theoretical literature on the multiple-field approach (Stemberger 2009, 2018c, 2022b).

Metzger's differentiation of self-awareness

Going forward with these considerations one might find helpful what Wolfgang Metzger says about the differentiation of the phenomenal world from the viewpoint of one's awareness: He distinguishes between self-awareness, awareness of one's "inner world" and awareness of one's "outer world":

"1. Self-awareness is to be understood as the awareness of the phenomenal, experienced ego (...). Awareness in this sense comprises in first place the simple awareness of one's own existence; secondly an already somewhat more differentiated awareness of one's state of mind; and finally, the very slowly developing awareness of one's own uniqueness, an awareness of one's enduring personality in its specificity, in being different from others, this being the true subject of self-knowledge (...).

The actual and unquestionable core of self-perception is certainly the awareness of one's state of mind: as the awareness of how one is at this moment, in what
mood one is, what one 'feels like'; in other words: the whole world of moods,
feelings, emotions and affects, intentions and aspirations, as one experiences and
feels them directly in himself. (...)

2 and 3. The two remaining areas of awareness or of the phenomenal world
are best understood in their mutual stand-off. They are, as I have said, the in-
ner-world consciousness, for the contents of which I have suggested the expression 'the envisioned,' (das Vorgestellte) and the outer-world consciousness, for the contents of which the expressions 'the encountered' (das
Angetroffene) or 'the encountering' (das Begegnende) seem to me most appropriate." (Metzger 1959, transl. from German)

Galli: Forms of Prägnanz in the ego-world-relationship

Finally, the contribution of the Italian Gestalt psychologist Giuseppe Galli
must be addressed. He has devoted a significant part of his life to the research of
the phenomenal self. In one of his major works, the "Psychologie der sozialen
Tugenden" (psychology of social virtues; Galli 2005) he discusses the phenomenology and dynamics of various social behaviors, or "modes of being together". This can be understood as Gestalt qualities of human relations or - as
Galli himself proposes - as "Forms of Prägnanz of relationship structures"
(Galli 2010, 58ff).

Galli explicates this in dealing with the "social virtues" of dedication, of gratitude, of wonder, of repentance and forgiveness, of trust, honesty, and hope. As
Galli shows, these "virtues" are not properties or traits of a person, but specific
forms of prägnant order of the psychological field, especially the structural and
functional integration of the phenomenal ego in his interpersonal environment
in concrete situations.

Galli continues with this analysis, what Max Wertheimer in his posthumously
published work "Productive Thinking" tried to demonstrate with his examples
"Two boys playing badminton" and "A young girl describes his office"
(Wertheimer 1945/2020). Wertheimer as well as Galli try to understand the structure and dynamics of the field, what factors determine the behavior of the phenomenal ego in his phenomenal world, in particular in relation to his fellow men.
So here we come full circle again in our brief review of Gestalt theoretical approaches to ego and self.

5. Basic Principles for Therapeutic Relationship and Practice in Gestalt Theoretical Psychotherapy

Angelika Böhm[23]

Gestalt Theoretical Psychotherapy (GTP) is legally recognized as a scientific psychotherapy method in its own right in Austria. The Gestalt theory of the Berlin School (Wertheimer, Köhler, Koffka and Lewin) also radiated into the psychotherapeutic field from the very beginnings. Early on, from the 1920ies, pioneering work was done on the Gestalt theoretical understanding of healthy and pathological development (cf. Stemberger 2002). Gestalt theory also influenced more or less directly the development of several psychotherapeutic schools, including Gestalt therapy, group psychoanalysis and other psychotherapeutic approaches focused on group dynamics, and later on catathymic-imaginative psychotherapy. As regards psychotherapeutic understanding and the existential needs of the person, Gestalt theory has much in common with both Adlerian individual psychology (cf. Soff & Ruh 1999) and with Carl Rogers' client-centered approach (cf. Metzger 1977). Also, some psychoanalytic schools of thought have sought to integrate Gestalt theoretical insights (cf. Waldvogel 1992; Galli 2017; Trombini & Trombini 2006).

A new attempt to formulate a Gestalt Theoretical Psychotherapy in a comprehensive and consistent way was made in the late 1970s in Germany, when Hans-Jürgen P. Walter published his doctoral thesis as a book under the title "Gestalttheorie und Psychotherapie" (Gestalt Theory and Psychotherapy; Walter 1985, 1994) and the *Society for Gestalt Theory and its Applications* (GTA) was founded, an international community that allowed psychotherapists to join forces with other people interested in the advancement of Gestalt theory in psychology and other fields of science and research. After a first phase in which the orientation in the psychotherapy section of this multidisciplinary community was more towards a Gestalt theoretical foundation of Gestalt therapy and related therapeutic methods, this approach increasingly developed

---

[23] Based on a lecture at the 21st Scientific Conference of the GTA "Motion – Spaces of Human Experience," 13th–15th June 2019, Warsaw, Poland, subsequently published in 2021 as an article in a special issue of the e-journal *Gestalt Theory*, 43(1), 69-86, here republished in a revised version. This contribution essentially follows the basic statements of the elaboration by Gerhard Stemberger, which was published in German in the journal *Phänomenal – Zeitschrift für Gestalttheoretische Psychotherapie* (Stemberger, 2018a; 2019a; 2019b). I sincerely thank the reviewers of my manuscript for their helpful suggestions; the remaining shortcomings of this paper remain entirely mine.

into an independent psychotherapy method in its own right, and with the claim of being an integrative approach. In this particular variant it has mainly gained a foothold in the German-speaking countries.

The purpose of this contribution is to present and justify the practice of Gestalt Theoretical Psychotherapy in its main features and more recent developments. While presentations of therapy methods and research often focus on what is practically done there, we want to take the top-down path in the Gestalt theoretical sense. In order to describe what actually happens in psychotherapy, it is necessary to understand the overarching whole in which it is embedded. The frame of reference in which the practical procedures in psychotherapy acquire their meaning and develop their effectiveness is the relationship between therapist and client in the particular therapeutic situation. (Stemberger 2018b).

There is a scientific consensus that the psychotherapeutic relationship has a significant influence on the outcome of a therapy. Since the beginnings of psychotherapy, aspects of relationship have played a central role. Orlinsky and Howard (1986) concluded based on the meta-analysis of over 2300 studies that the quality of the therapeutic relationship is of central importance for the therapeutic outcome. This result was subsequently confirmed by numerous studies (e.g., Horvath & Symonds 1991; Strunk & Schiepek 2014). No finding of psychotherapy research has been validated as frequently as the correlation between the effect factor quality of therapy relationship and the success of psychotherapy (Pfammatter et al. 2012). This correlation can be demonstrated across different therapeutic procedures, such as psychodynamic and cognitive-behavioral approaches (Flückiger et al., 2015; Barwinski, 2014). For therapeutic interventions to be effective, they must be embedded in a good working relationship, since therapeutic relationship is the basis of psychotherapy (Strunk & Schiepek 2014).

Accepting the factual duplication of the psychotherapeutic situation and building on it

A Gestalt theoretical approach to the psychotherapeutic relationship first considers the epistemological background. From the point of view of critical realism, it cannot be assumed that we have only *one* single therapeutic relationship and *one* single therapeutic situation. In fact, when we talk about therapy, we have *two* therapeutic relationships and *two* therapeutic situations. The therapeutic relationship involves one experience in the phenomenal world *of the client,* and one experience in the phenomenal world *of the therapist* (cf. Sternek 2021; Stemberger 2013).

The therapeutic relationship in the client's phenomenal world is not the same as the therapeutic relationship in the therapist's phenomenal world. Although generally there will be similarities in certain areas, there will often also be significant differences in other respects. Between these worlds understanding and reciprocity is possible, but not always given in advance. Therapeutic practice must take this into account (Stemberger 2018b).

"So, what happens in the therapeutic field of the therapist's phenomenal world is by no means identical with what happens in the therapeutic field of the client's phenomenal world. It has first to become a fact in the world of the other to become a field part there, and it will then function as a part of this other field, possibly differing considerably from how it functions as part of the therapist's field." (Trombini et al. 2019, p. 64)

Understanding and agreement between these two worlds are basically possible. More than that, they are necessary for a successful therapy process. What matters is the creation of a psychological contact between these two phenomenal worlds, which only succeeds if it is supported by communicative processes. Experience and perception of both worlds should correspond to some extent (Stemberger 2019a).

In this sense, research on the topic of therapeutic relationships can only be read with a certain skepticism from a Gestalt theoretical point of view, where they report *one* therapeutic relationship. The nature of the therapeutic relationship can never be viewed adequately only from within the therapist's phenomenal world or from within the client's phenomenal world; so it should always be clearly stated which of the two one is speaking about or investigating. Although client and therapist "factors" influencing the working alliance are identified in the research concepts by interviewing therapists and clients alike (Horvath & Luborsky 1993; Norcross & Lambert 2018), their results still very often refer to a fictitious single and uniform therapeutic relationship.

The Nature of the Therapeutic Relationship

A special working alliance aimed at psychotherapeutically supporting the client in overcoming a particular state of mental suffering, emotional distress, or psychic restriction is seen in GTP as an essential part of the therapeutic relationship. Like any relationship, it is a genuine encounter between people and therefore cannot be limited to the aspect of a working alliance. As Wolfgang Metzger described in 2001 in general – not psychotherapy related – terms (62ff), a therapeutic relationship possesses Gestalt qualities, with properties of material (*Materialeigenschaften*), properties of structure (*Struktureigenschaften*) and properties of essence (or expressive properties; *Wesenseigenschaften*): The properties of "material" are mainly determined by the persons involved (their age, sex, and other "material" properties), the structural properties result mainly from the particularities of the coming together in a therapy and its course, which structure the relationship in a specific way. The expressive properties of the relationship – whether tense, trusting, insecure, confusing, etc. – will change over and over during the course of therapy and, above all, will not always mainifest themselves in the same way on both sides (therapist and client). A therapeutic relationship also shows other Gestalt qualities: On the one hand, it is not static, but rather a progressive Gestalt (*Verlaufsgestalt*), and on the other hand it is characterized by dynamic auto-organizing tendencies (Stemberger 2018b)[24].

Therapeutic relationships can be more or less *prägnant* (concise). Giuseppe Galli analyzed social virtues that are important not only for the psychotherapeutic relationship, but for all interpersonal encounters. These social virtues are *Prägnanz* forms (conciseness forms) of relational structures (Galli 2005; 2017). Stemberger noted: "When we think of relationships in which one person tries to help another, nurtures or supports the other in a therapeutic way, and the other person receives help, accepts care, and accepts the therapeutic options, then, in the successful case, all the social virtues analyzed by Giuseppe Galli take effect on both sides." (2020b, 44; transl. AB)

The social virtues analyzed by Galli (devotion, gratitude, wonder, repentance, trust and sincerity), as well as their psychological contrasts (escape into fantasy, envy and presumption, obtrusiveness and possessiveness, insincerity, indifference and contempt), can come to light in the treatment of the client's relationships in his/her everyday life, but they can also reveal themselves as *Prägnanz* forms of the therapeutic relationship. On the part of the therapist, the *Prägnanz* form of devotion can be seen as the basic form of the psychotherapeutic situation – in the sense of one's devotion to addressing the therapeutic concerns of the client (Stemberger 2013).

Threefold Relationship Centering in GTP

Not only the therapeutic relationship, but relationships in general play an important role in GTP, particularly as the human being is regarded as a genuine social being. The phenomenal world of a person is a social world in which he/she is in close interaction with fellow beings and with human communities. The human being is thus not seen as an individual being to which social references are added only later, but as a primarily social being whose experience

---

[24] With Luccio (1993, 2003), we prefer the term "auto-organization" to that of "self-organization" to avoid conflations with concepts that assume a "self" as the organizer of such processes that actually do not require an "organizer".

and behavior is determined by the relationship between the person and his/her environment – and there again above all by his/her fellow human beings. This phenomenal world is therefore not seen as an isolated individual social world. With his/her behavior, a person influences the phenomenal worlds of his/her fellow human beings, which in turn can lead to corresponding reactions. In addition, it is also a world socially shaped by the respective concrete socio-economic circumstances, gender fate, power and politics (cf. Zabransky et al. 2018).

In this sense, GTP considers itself to be a relationship-centered approach in which the therapist's attention is essentially focused on the client's relationships. On the one hand the particular interest lies in the relationships the client has with his/her fellow human beings (e.g., family, love and friendship relationships, relationships in work-life and in cultural and political associations), on the other hand also in the relationship between therapist and client in the respective therapeutic situation, and finally also in the relationship the client has with him- or herself. These three stages or spheres of relationships interact closely with each other: Sometimes problems and coping opportunities that the client has in his/her everyday relationships manifest in the therapeutic relationship, perhaps in a somewhat modified form. This special type of "transference" offers the opportunity for such problems to be dealt with directly on the spot (on the Gestalt theoretical concept of "transference": cf. Kästl 2007). In the protected environment of the therapeutic situation, one may try out new forms of dealing with these difficult and challenging situations. When successful, new experiences of relationship-healing may be found in the therapeutic encounter (Stemberger 2018b).

As the American Gestalt psychologist Mary Henle has shown in her study of the phenomenology of personality, there is also a close correlation between the nature and expression of a person's relationship to his/her fellow human beings and his/her relationship to him- or herself (Henle 1962; Stemberger 2010b). A focus on the client's relationship to him- or herself, including its manifold interactions with relationships to other people and groups in everyday life and with his/her relationship to his/her therapist, can only succeed if the therapist has also investigated these interactions within him-/herself. This threefold relationship-centered GTP can finally be expressed in the fact that the therapist considers it an essential therapeutic goal and at the same time an indicator for the therapy's progress to support the client's various relationships in their development towards more positive forms and higher levels of conciseness/Prägnanz (Stemberger 2018b).

Therapeutic Attitude

The meaning of the German wording 'therapeutische Haltung' is closely related to both 'therapeutic attitude' and 'therapeutic stance'. In literature both designations are used depending on the focus (Jørgensen, 2019). This contribution refers to those aspects of the therapist's attitude towards his/her tasks, the way of encounter with his/her clients and to the fundamental orientation towards psychotherapeutic work in GTP, which is why the term attitude seems more appropriate in this context.

Several researchers have found that the therapeutic attitude varies considerably from one therapist to the other and confirmed that the therapeutic attitude is closely related to the epistemological background and theoretical orientation of the different therapeutic schools (e.g., Taubner et al. 2010; Sandell et al. 2006). In Gestalt Theoretical Psychotherapy, with its special characteristic that its conception is not primarily based on a certain praxeology or doctrine of disease, but explicitly on the epistemological position of critical realism, the therapeutic attitude is aligned accordingly. It considers the different experiences of different people, the need to respect different phenomenal realms and distinguishes itself from monopersonal approaches (cf. Sternek 2021).

The course of the psychotherapy process is essentially determined by the quality of the therapeutic relationship, which is shaped on the therapist's side by a certain attitude towards his/her task, his/her client and him-/herself. From the very first encounter between client and therapist, as in all subsequent encounters, the relationship that develops between them is expressed in the attitude with which they face each other and will relate to each other in the future. "This attitude is both the manifestation and the core of their relationship with each other." (Stemberger 2019a, 29; transl. AB)

Such attitudes arise "internally" from the attitudes of the person concerned towards him-/herself and towards the other person and towards therapy, from the expectations and readiness associated with these attitudes and how they are brought into the encounter and cooperation. "Externally" this attitude can also become visible in their posture, in their gestures and "rituals", in all aspects of their interaction with each other. Here, too, it is not only about the therapist's attitude towards the client, but also about the therapist's attitude towards him-/herself and at least towards his or her task.

Gestalt Theoretical Psychotherapy is characterized by certain ideas about the attitude in which the therapist should encounter his/her client and the therapeutic task. The therapist's main requirement is an attitude of "objectivity", which means that one should not be guided in therapy by selfish personal interests, but by the "demands of the situation". This attitude has its origin in the social virtue of devotion described by Giuseppe Galli – an attitude of human respect (Stemberger, ibid.).

As regards the question of what constitutes a healing encounter in psychotherapy, there is a close agreement with the findings of Carl Rogers, who formulated six necessary and sufficient conditions for personality development through psychotherapy:

"For therapy to occur it is necessary that these conditions exist.

1. That two persons are in *contact*.

2. That the first person, whom we shall term the client, is in a state of *incongruence*, being *vulnerable*, or *anxious*.

3. That the second person, whom we shall term the therapist, is *congruent* in the *relationship*.

4. That the therapist is *experiencing unconditional positive regard* toward the client.

5. That the therapist is *experiencing* an *empathic* understanding of the client's *internal frame of reference*.

6. That the client *perceives*, at least to a minimal degree, conditions 4 and 5, the *unconditional positive regard of* the therapist for him, and the *empathic* understanding of the therapist." (Rogers, 1959, p. 213; emphasis in original)

These conditions, which unfortunately are often reduced to three "therapist variables" in the psychotherapy literature (congruence, unconditional positive regard and empathy), do justice to the relationship character of psychotherapy in a way that coincides with the viewpoint of critical-realism as to the psychotherapeutic situation.

They point to the fact that the therapist and client do not live in a common phenomenal world, but each in his/her own. In both worlds a phenomenal therapist and a phenomenal client meet each other. A client-therapist encounter is experienced in the phenomenal world of both the client and the therapist, but how that encounter is experienced can and does differ significantly between the phenomenal worlds of the client and the therapist. Through processes of mutual perception, communication and behavior, despite this difference, or even because of this difference, in the phenomenal worlds of both persons involved, a genuine interpersonal relationship can come about that sufficiently agrees and sufficiently differs.

The important thing now is that a psychological contact between these two worlds develops. This succeeds wherever an agreement between these two worlds can be achieved through communicative processes. Congruence, positive regard and empathy on the part of the therapist therefore only make sense if they are also present in the phenomenal world of the client (Stemberger 2019a).

One of the guiding principles of the Gestalt Theoretical Psychotherapy is that the therapeutic situation should act as a "place of creative freedom" for both sides and should be shaped accordingly (Walter 1985; derived from Metzger 1962/2022). Creative freedom therefore means to cope with one's own individuality as well as with the individuality of one's counterpart. According to Metzger, sustainable changes can only be achieved on the basis of a person's inner forces. Arbitrary, enforced changes to living beings or living processes from outside are in the best case ineffective, in the worst case they are acts of ruthlessness or even violence. In this sense, the therapist will not take a "making" attitude in which he or she sets the pace of work and the topics.

The Therapy Situation as a Place of Creative Freedom

With Metzger we assume that the possibilities for the development of the inner forces are given in the human being. These forces do not have to be formed by the therapist first, but his or her task is to create the conditions under which such forces can occur and to remove obstacles so that, where they exist, they can come into operation – with the aim that something special, new, peculiar, original, genuine, true can emerge, like clarification of unexpected connections, a discovery or invention, or an unexpected and convincing solution to a problem. Creative freedom does not mean the freedom to do anything, but the freedom to do what is right in a particular situation (Metzger 1962, 75; 2022, 60). This kind of freedom is not seen in the sense of being free from arbitrariness or from external restrictions and specifications, it is seen in the sense of being free from internal and external barriers and forces that distract from the actual goal. What is right for the client in a given situation does not depend on the therapist's assessment, but neither does it simply depend on the client's assessment. Doubts or conflicts about what the situation is and what to do have finally led the client into therapy. What is at stake, then, is helping the client find a clearer understanding of the situation and what it requires of him. The therapist lends him his skills for this search, not his own opinion as the determining one.

Metzger (1962, 18ff; 2022, 12ff) has detailed six "characteristics of working at the living" (living beings and living processes) as those conditions under which creative forces can develop and unfold. These characteristics were applied to the psychotherapeutic field by Walter (1977). These characteristics do not only refer to psychotherapeutic situations, they come into play everywhere where one has to do with living beings (such as in upbringing, care, in education, even in connection with animals and plants). The leading principle is "reverence" for the inner qualities of the person, which is understood as a self-regulating system (Galli 2007). Due to their interdisciplinary significance, these characteristics are also increasingly gaining recognition outside Gestalt Theoretical Psychotherapy, for example in educational sciences (Soff 2018) and humanistic therapy methods (Kriz 2014).

In the following, the six characteristics, as developed by Metzger and applied by Walter (1985) to psychotherapy, will be briefly described:

1. Non-Exchangeability of Forms

Nothing may be imposed on a living being that is contrary to its nature. Likewise, only those potentials can be brought to maturity that are inherent in a person or a living being. Metzger explained this fact by means of the difference to dead (non-living) material (such as a work piece made of gypsum, clay or metal), which one can produce, craft or make anything with it – just as he or she likes, just when he or she likes, just as he or she wants it to be. In connection with living beings, in the long run, one cannot force anything which is against their nature. Only that which is inherent in the living being as a possibility can be brought to an unfolding. This is not to say that it would be impossible to impose anything on a person from the outside. But this possibility is considered to be very limited and not permanent and contradicts man's disposition to auto-organization.

2. Shaping the Process by Using the Forces Inherent within the Living Being

Metzger described this characteristic vaguely translated as "shaping from inherent forces". The impulses and forces that realize the desired form have their origin in the cared-for being. The psychotherapist is challenged to set conducive surrounding conditions and to strengthen or weaken these inner forces at certain points, so that they satisfy the needs in the current situation. Therefore, psychotherapy will only succeed when it is respectful of the indwelling forces within the client. Each psychotherapy situation needs to be adjusted to the individual possibilities and abilities of both human parts – in an interactive process between the psychotherapist and the client. Any procedures executed along a standardized pattern, irrespective of the individual and the situational needs, are out of place. The psychotherapist rather has to stay in close contact with a given situation and with the client's skills as well as his or her own skills or faculties in order to find those paths of discovery which are innate in this individual.

3. Non-Exchangeability of Working Times

Every living being, especially every human being, has its own time and moments which are particularly fruitful for change. Not any given time or point of psychotherapy is suitable for every procedure and every step taken thereafter. Planned procedures do not mean that the psychotherapist follows a rigid pattern without questioning whether the time is right for the client to take certain steps or undergo certain procedures. Every person has his/her own productive times for discovery and change. A Gestalt-theoretical psychotherapist does not determine the exact course of the development steps in advance.

4. Non-Exchangeability of Working Speed

In this context, it is also impossible to specify the speed of operation or speed of working. It cannot be arbitrarily accelerated or slowed down. Sometimes the therapist has to wait patiently, because no one can "do growing". And as it is sometimes necessary to wait for the right time, it is then an obligation for the therapist to really seize the opportunity.

5. Accepting Detours

Sometimes the therapist has to accept detours, because clients do not always go straight to their defined goal. Therapists will often have to tolerate diversions, or to even make provisions for them deliberately, when they have realized that there are indispensable intermediary steps in the client's unfolding discovery process. Here, trust in self-regulation plays an important role.

6. Mutuality of influence

All things that happen in the psychotherapeutic process influence one another. There's reciprocity of everything that goes on. Psychotherapy is a collaborative process, a joint process of discovery and change within a vital relational situation occurring between two (or more) humans. Any occurrence is to be comprehended as a field process that complies with the rules of the psychic field. "Although geared towards the clarification of a situation, of the developmental potential and the need of support by *one certain* person, with the professional help of the *other*, both do affect each other, opening themselves to this interaction and adopting an egalitarian attitude, which they use mindfully and consciously for the clarification to be achieved." (Stemberger 2008, 100).

All these characteristics specify the necessary conditions for the development of self-regulation. For the psychotherapist, it is the observance of these characteristics that is paramount, not the use of certain techniques or forms of intervention (Kästl, 2011). The same applies to the "social virtues" described by Giuseppe Galli. The attitudes and behavior patterns in therapy anchored in such insights therefore not only claim to do justice to the nature of human beings and the concrete encounter situation in psychotherapy, but also to lend effectiveness to therapy by promoting the self-healing powers of human beings (Stemberger 2019b). With Galli (2017), we speak of Gestalt theory as a "school of respect".

Forms of Encounter and Cooperation

In explaining working at the living, Metzger distinguished three basic forms of this work, which parallel the leadership styles described and examined by Lewin, Lippitt & White (1939). He described *care, leadership* and *fight* as three basic forms which in practical work often complement, mix and merge (Metzger 1962/2022). Kästl (2011) emphasizes these three basic forms as valid for psychotherapeutic work, as well as for all professional and private relationships we engage in in our daily lives: In terms of psychotherapeutic work Kästl summarizes as follows: Care means that the client's will is at the forefront of the joint approach and the therapist remains largely in the background, consciously allowing himself to be guided by the client's concerns. This type of encounter will be particularly necessary if the client is emotionally strongly involved in a topic to be worked on, needing nothing more than the sustained interest and receptiveness of the therapist – when more active participation, beyond caring support, could disturb the process.

As regards the second form (leading), one's own sphere of will is expanded by including the will of another person. In addition to the therapist's own will, the client's will must therefore be preserved. Therapist and client pursue a common goal, whereby the client willingly leaves the therapist in charge, which results from the mere fact that the client comes into treatment and confides in the therapist's expertise. In the third form, the fight, the will of the other person is overcome in a concrete context, in extreme cases even broken. The latter may occur in rare situations in psychotherapeutic processes, when the patient endangers himself or herself or others. Here a maximum of transparency is required on the part of the therapist in order to dissolve the fight as quickly as possible and return to leadership as a form of relationship.

Stemberger (2019a) adds that these three basic forms are not limited to the therapist, but also take place on the client's side. Both do this with each other or in relation to each other, whereby it can become clear in what way the client cares, leads and fights in his everyday life relationships, but also how he cares, leads and fights in dealing with himself. In addition, he states that this caring, leading and fighting must be embedded in another, overarching form of encounter: *cooperation* between client and therapist in the pursuit of the client's concerns. For this it is necessary that both agree from the beginning that the therapist will also be involved and available as a reliable partner at eye level.

Working Procedures and Methods

"Practicing phenomenology" together by therapist and client, combined with a change activating force field analysis, are the fundamental working methods of GTP. While practicing phenomenology is aimed at "looking at what is" as unreservedly as possible, at what the client directly encountered finds in her or his phenomenal world, the force field analysis aims to find out – by experimenting and varying – the forces that decisively determine how this phenomenal world is found and how it works ("discovering what forces are at work") (cf. Zabransky et al. 2018).

The phenomenal world of the client cannot be explored by the therapist, but only by the client him- / herself, because he or she alone has immediate access to his or her own phenomenal world (Stemberger 2016). The therapist can only learn about it through the client. In doing so the therapist encourages the client to seriously engage with her or his experience and the thoughts and ideas associated with it and to share these in a dialogical process with the therapist. While the client is to become his/her own diagnostician, it is the task of the therapist to accompany this exploration competently and unselfishly (Stemberger 2019b). This should be as unaffected as possible by presumptions and reservations. In this context, Stemberger (2016) emphasizes that what is "discovered", which simply has to be "accepted as it is", refers not only to what is descriptively encountered in the experience, such as what is seen, heard, felt and sensed, but also to what is thought, imagined, remembered and planned. "This way of working is based on trusting that the simple recognition and acknowledgement of 'what is' forms the basic prerequisite for any problem solving and healing". (Stemberger 2019b, 40; transl. AB)

Practicing phenomenology jointly with the client always includes the force field analysis. It is not only about understanding and deepening the client's experience, but also about getting to the bottom of the effective driving and inhibiting forces, so that the emergence of the phenomenally encountered facts can be understood. These forces are, on the client's side, his/her own needs, plans and goals and the obstacles effective in the internal personal area, as regards his/her experienced environment and his/her interrelation with it, the requirements from this environment and the associated inhibiting and promoting forces and induced needs and goals; finally, as a framework condition that defines the potential space of all these forces, the material, non-psychological conditions of the person's existence (e.g., gender, age, social class affiliation or physiological condition). In doing so, the therapist encourages his or her client to check the assumptions and convictions about him-/herself in the here and now of the therapy situation by inviting him or her to try out variations of the corresponding situation (e.g., to assume a position of power, a different time perspective, etc.). Such an experimentally varying procedure (Luchins & Luchins 1959; Lindorfer, Luchins & Luchins 2020) can, if successful, not only promote new insights but also create a new psychological situation itself. In this sense we speak of change-activating force field analysis.

Practicing phenomenology and force field analysis take place situation-focused "top down". The "top" or "the whole" is understood here as: The psychological situation the client is currently in; the person of the client in interaction with his or her environment; the therapeutic relationship – as basis for the next concrete steps to be taken. In any case, the Gestalt-theoretical psychotherapist does not proceed in such a way that individual symptoms or personality areas are researched and "worked on" one after the other and independently of each other in order to form a summative image of the overall situation or of the client's person, but conversely always tries to start from a view of the client's overall psychological situation, in which individual problems, personality traits, balance of power etc. are embedded. "It is the character of the psychological situation as a whole that determines the peculiarity of individual parts, not the reverse." (Zabransky et al. 2018, 160; transl. AB) For this reason, interventions and techniques in GTP must always be right for the client's overall psychological situation and must also be within the range of the therapist's capabilities.

Practicing phenomenology and force field analysis are applied in an emotion-focused and insight-oriented manner. GTP assumes that for a way out of mental crises and disorders the human being also needs insight into his/her situation and possibilities and that psychotherapy must support him/her in gaining and implementing such insights. Insight-oriented problem analysis, as developed by Erna Hruschka (1969) based on Gestalt theoretical research, is regarded as a comprehensive Gestalt process that can lead to necessary restructuring. Emotions play a decisive role in this process, as numerous studies (especially by Kurt Lewin and his students) indicate. In GTP emotions are seen as Prägnanz forms of experiencing oneself in the world and experiencing oneself to this world. They concisely express the needs and goals of a person (cf. Stemberger & Sternek 2019). In emotions and feeling it is prägnant (concise) in a holistic way who you are in which world and what results directly from it. Therefore, the Gestalt-theoretical psychotherapist preferentially directs the attention to the experience of emotions and promotes the expression of emotions both with the client and with oneself – not for the sake of an end in itself or to relieve tension, but as a natural part of clarification processes.

Given its epistemological allegiance to critical realism, which itself invites both phenomenology and a relationship-centered approach, the therapeutic process of GTP is strongly dialogical. There is need to attend not only to communication between therapist and client, but the way client relates to his/her world, both fellow human beings and communities contained therein, but the client's internal communications – the "inner dialogue" between different "parts", "aspects" or psychological functions of a person.

When the therapeutic process is no longer primarily about discovering new insights, but rather about consolidating and optimizing existing or newly acquired abilities and skills, GTP proceeds in a practicing and experimenting manner. Consistent with Gestalt theory, practicing is not understood as mechanical repetition, but rather as experimentation with previous attainments aimed at further developing and honing them, under new, more differentiated conditions (Stemberger 2019b).

Forms of Interventions and Techniques

Regarding techniques and methods, GTP is open to diverse forms of work from different areas, if they reflect the particular demands of the situation (*Gefordertheit der Lage*) and align with Gestalt theoretical principles. GTP rejects the uncritical embrace of evidence-based treatment in nomothetic contexts, whose "one-size-fits-all," cookbook approaches may be insufficiently attuned to individual needs and differences. Contrary to the medical model, successful psychotherapy cannot be measured by specific methods for specific disorders. Instead, the therapeutic process as a whole is decisive (Norcross & Wampold 2011; Lambert 2013). From the point of view of GTP, the use of techniques plays only a subordinate and supporting role. Whether a particular technique is used depends less on the specificity of the form of intervention than the therapeutic situation and therapeutic relationship in which it is embedded.

GTP regards the human being as an open system that is permanently self-regulating. The process of self-regulation is directed by the phenomenal world of a person, powered by his or her needs and quasi-needs (*Quasi-Bedürfnisse*) (Metzger 1969 in 1986). From the beginning of their lives, people actively interact in and with their environment, seeking both balance and new experiences. Accordingly, the experienced, phenomenal world is a dynamic system that constantly strives for new states of equilibrium (*Fließgleichgewicht*). Following the findings of Gestalt theoretical research, this self-regulation is subject to the laws of Gestalt, which are applied here in the sense of the Prägnanz principle (cf. Köhler 1957/1993; Rausch 1966; Luccio 2019). The task of GTP is now to help people whose lives have become overly unbalanced to find a new dynamic balance, to the greatest degree possible. Interventions and techniques should be aimed at supporting reorganization and restructuring tendencies that are already indwelling as demands in the phenomenal world of the client.

Stemberger (2019b) enumerates the different forms and techniques of intervention that GTP employs to achieve therapeutic objectives:

1. Forms of intervention and techniques that may induce certain changes in the client's systems of tension, i.e., directly address his needs and plans.

The effect of conscious and unconscious needs, objectives and meanings will have to be examined in order to be able to establish or maintain tension systems, if necessary, or, in the case of tension systems that are no longer appropriate, to promote their conversion or reduction. Verbal and non-verbal forms of intervention range from directing attention to one's own aspirations (e.g. with the question "What do you want right now?") or the aspirations of others ("What do they want from you right now?"), to trying out the effect of expressing these aspirations, to forms that make the currently effective needs and aspirations in their various aspects directly experienceable (e.g. in fantasies of wish fulfillment, in imagined staging, in dialogical works, etc.). Current unconscious aspirations can be rendered accessible by directing attention to posture, body movements, the sound of the voice or the melody of speech, for example. Possible conflicting or contradictory aspirations can thus be uncovered.

2. Forms of intervention and techniques which may induce structural changes in the client's life space.

Referring to Kurt Lewin's field theory, a distinction can be made between verbal and non-verbal forms of intervention

* which are able to induce an extension or reduction of the time dimension of the life space (e.g. moment exercises, time travel, life panorama, etc.),

* which are able to induce a change in the degree of reality of the life space (or parts thereof), e.g. transformation of the experienced into a film scene, magic and the like,

* which are able to induce a higher or lower differentiation of the life space (e.g. viewing through a magnifier or telescope),

* which are able to induce liquefaction or solidification of the life space (or parts thereof),

* which are able to induce extension or narrowing of the life space,

* which are able to induce a change in the degree of order.

Although most of the forms of intervention listed here mostly focus on one of these dimensions, their impact also affects more or less all the others.

3. Forms of intervention and techniques that focus on the tension systems and structures in the therapeutic relationship.

On the one hand, the therapeutic relationship can be addressed as a learning field, on the other hand as "transference" and "countertransference" events. The forms of intervention require a particularly sensitive approach and range from simply addressing the current relationship or proceedings, to clarifying relationships in dialogue, to techniques in which the situation-determining relationship in the perception of the therapist becomes the subject of therapy.

4. Forms of intervention and techniques that focus on the tension systems and structures in other social relations of the client.

A distinction is made here between those interventions which explore the conditions for the emergence of ego-centered experiencing and behavior, and such which promote situation-centered experiencing and behavior. This category includes all verbal and non-verbal interventions and techniques that are suitable to convey the client into the experience of different situations (of the present, the past or the future).

The differentiation between these four functional basic forms of interventions and techniques is primarily conceptual with a focus on aim and effect. In practice, they mostly overlap. A wide variety of forms of intervention can now be assigned to these categories, which can be used in GTP depending on the situation and the requirements.

6. "The way you make me feel" – Feeling-causality in language communication

Andrzej Żuczkowski & Gerhard Stemberger[25]

Summary:

"You make me angry" - "You make me happy": in such formulations a whole world full of strange relationships and distributions of power is revealed - usually quite unnoticed, but all the more effective. In the first part of this article, Andrzej Żuczkowski explores the background and theoretical explanations for this peculiar world, based on memories of his encounter with this topic during his Transactional Analysis training. His analysis is mainly based on considerations and findings of the Belgian experimental psychologist Albert Michotte (1881-1965), whose name is inseparably connected with the research of "phenomenal causality", and of Wolfgang Metzger. Gerhard Stemberger concludes by addressing the viewpoint that determines the understanding and handling of the phenomena of naïve feeling-causality in Gestalt Theoretical Psychotherapy.

[1] Introduction

When I (Andrzej Żuczkowski) began my training in Transactional Analysis psychotherapy in the '80s, one of the first things I learned by direct experience during my personal analysis was that nobody can make me feel good or bad and that I cannot make someone else feel good or bad. For example, when I used sentences like "my wife makes me feel angry" I was confronted by my psychotherapist, who, among other things, told me that there is no cause-effect relationship between what a person says (verbal action) or does (non-verbal action, behaviour) and what I feel: nobody has the power to make me feel good or bad, unless I want. In other words, no one except myself can make me feel good or bad.

Accepting this point of view took a long time and a deep personal change because, before my training, I was firmly convinced of the opposite point of view, i.e., that I can make others feel good or bad and that others can make me feel good or bad. Who has direct experience of group psychotherapy knows how much such a belief is spread over, deep-rooted, strongly defended, and how obvious and natural it appears to those who share it. Such a 'common sense' belief, implied in sentences like "my wife makes me feel angry", can be considered as a real *causal theory of interpersonal relationships*, for it explains how the relationships among people function. Since such a causal theory is about feelings, emotions, affects and the like, it can be called a theory of 'feeling-causality'.

---

[25] A German version of this article appeared 2019 in the journal *Phänomenal*, *11*(2), 3-20, under the title: "Wer uns die Gefühle macht".

I accepted this kind of psychotherapeutic point of view since for me it was liberating (from symbiotic confusions, etc.) as compared to the other one, the 'common sense' point of view.

Anyway, at the scientific level, I was not completely satisfied with the arguments, though logical and rational, which psychotherapists gave me in support of their point of view. I looked for in the relevant literature among those psychotherapeutic theories that share the same point of view as Transactional Analysis (Neuro-Linguistic Programming, Perl's Gestalt therapy, etc.), but I did not find any satisfying argument.

In addition to this 'scientific un-satisfaction', I had some more unanswered questions running in my head: supposing that the psychotherapeutic point of view is scientifically valid, grounded, why in everyday talk do speakers *use* sentences implying affective causality in such a normal and spontaneous, non-problematic way, and why do they *believe* in the underlying theory of feeling-causality so strongly? How and why did such a belief originate and take root? In other terms, if such sentences are not scientifically grounded, why did they impose in everyday talk and still keep on imposing?

Since in the '80s I was (and still I am) an experimental Gestalt psychologist as well, I tried to answer the above-mentioned un-satisfaction and questions from a Gestalt theoretical point of view (Zuczkowski 1995, Chapter 7; 1998, 1999, 2004, 2008) and presented my ideas in a workshop during the 14th International GTA Conference in Graz (2005).

The second author of this article, Gerhard Stemberger, also participated in this workshop. At a meeting in Macerata in 2018, we came to talk about this workshop in Graz and the whole topic and realized that it still seems very important to us. From my earlier work and subsequent discussions with Gerhard Stemberger, the joint article now at hand emerged.

This paper mainly tries to give answers to the following questions:

(1) How can the everyday use of formulations implying this kind of causal theory of the origin of feelings be explained? How can the belief in feeling causality underlying them be explained from a Gestalt theoretical point of view, with special reference to W. Metzger's modes of appeal ('Anmutungsweisen') and to Albert Michotte's experiments on causality perception?

(2) How do phenomena of perceived and believed feeling-causation between two persons occur in psychotherapies and how can they be understood and addressed in the psychotherapeutic context from the perspective of Gestalt Theoretical Psychotherapy?

[2] Feeling-Causality

In everyday talk speakers normally use sentences of the following types:

(1) "This movie *is amusing* me", "What they told him *saddened* him", "I'll *calm* her by telling her that she is right", "Their sudden departure *astonishes* me", "He *scared* me", etc.

(2) "You (or they/she/he/it) make(s) me *feel* angry (or sad/glad/happy…)".

(3) "She has an irritating habit; "His behaviour is *disgusting*; "They had a *depressing* defeat"; "You are a *fascinating* woman", etc.

In the above sentences, the verbs, verbal expressions and adjectives in italics are used to describe the effects, consequences, results that somebody or something has on somebody else's feelings, emotions, affects, moods, whatever they may be called. Though such sentences have a different syntactic structure, yet they share the same *causal* semantic structure which can be schematized in the following way: somebody or something (=A) causes, caused or will cause a certain feeling or emotion in somebody else (=B): anger, sadness, joy, boredom, astonishment, happiness, amusement…

We are dealing here with A's "causation", "production" "generation", "creation" of something new in B: a feeling, an emotion. For that reason, this kind of causation can be called *feeling causation* or *feeling-causality*.

[3] An implicit theory of interpersonal relations: The common sense or naïve point of view

For the above reasons, sentences of type (1)-(3) *are not simply ways of speaking*, they also *show what people believe* (think, are convinced) happens in language communication, i.e., they convey an implicit, underlying theory of interpersonal relations, common sense, confirmed and reinforced every day by the language itself.

As an example, let us suppose that after you have said or done something to me, I feel angry, and I tell you:

(4) "You make me feel angry".

By this utterance I mean it is you who aroused my anger; because of what you said to me, I got angry. I also mean that, if you had not said to me what you did or if you had said something different, I would not have got angry.

In this way, I attribute some effects which are inside me, internal to me (i.e., my feeling), to some causes which are outside me, external to me (i.e., your words and you). Such an attribution implies my firm belief that after your words I had no other way to react except that of feeling angry.[26]

In some contexts, besides my thinking of you as the one who caused those effects, I can also attribute to you the intention of and the responsibility for

---

[26] For the causal attribution theory see, in the Gestalt theoretical field, Heider 1958, in particular his psychology of common sense and naïve analysis of action.

having caused these effects. My "attributive reasoning" can then be paraphrased in the following way: (1) I feel angry (the effect) because (2) you made me feel angry by saying what you said (the causal link between your words and my anger); therefore (3) you intended to make me feel angry (intention) and you succeeded in doing so (responsibility).

[4] Focus on A

Example (4), as well as sentences of type (1) – (3), solves in a causal way the problem concerning the relations between A, what s/he says and B: it is A who causes, by saying what s/he says, B's anger.

To illustrate this point, it might be useful to refer to Metzger's (2001, Chapter V; 1975[3], Chapter V) notion of *Zentrierung* (Centering), i.e. the *hierarchical organization* (structure, order) *inside perceptual configurations*[27] :

Within the communication structure which is made up of A, his/her words and B, the whole focus is put on A and on what s/he says: B's effects are caused by A's words and then, after all, by A who utters them. The main role is given to A and to his/her words; s/he makes all the job: it is s/he who is the only one who acts, is active, performs an action, a verbal action, while B seems to be passive and dependent on what A says. Example (4), as well as sentences (1)-(3), does not acknowledge any autonomy to B but envision a whole dependence of B on A: B is wholly dependent on A.

Applying Metzger's terminology to communication structure, we could say that the organization inside the communication Gestalt, which includes at least three absolutely *necessary parts* ['Hauptteile'] (A, what s/he says and B), is totally *unbalanced* on one side, on A's side; the *weight, relief* and *emphasis* ['Gewichtsverteilung' and 'Schwerpunktlage'] are given to A and his/her words. A is the *phenomenal anchorage* of the communication Gestalt and the *principal direction* goes from A to B.

In our view, this causal structure centred on A would fall within what Metzger (2001, Chapter I) calls *naïve realism*. From the naïve point of view, as seen above, it is proper to state and believe that *A makes B feel angry*, i.e. that *A and his/her words cause B's anger*. Now the question is: is it proper to state and have such a belief also from the Gestalt theoretical point of view, i.e., from the point of view of what Metzger calls *critical realism*? In more general terms, *can* indeed somebody or something cause a feeling in somebody else? Is that really

---

[27] See in particular the notions of „Haupt- und Nebenteile, unentbehrliche und überflüssige Teile, tragenden und getragenen Bestandteile, Hauptrichtung, Verankerungspunkt, usw." (= principal and secondary, necessary and unnecessary, carrying and carried parts; principal directions and anchorage, etc.).

possible? If so, in which *critical*, not naïve, *sense* do we have to intend the notion of *cause*?

[5] Paradoxical consequences of feeling-causality

If I believe that my feelings are caused by what others said to me, then I grant myself no power over my feelings and so I do not take upon myself the responsibility for them; therefore, I am not in charge of them.

I attribute power and responsibility to others: it is you who make me feel the way I feel. Vice versa, I can cause other people's feelings and have power over them; I can control them and take charge of them.

If such were the case, I would be the cause of and the one responsible for your feelings but not my own; you would be the cause of and the one responsible for my feelings but not your own. Each of us would be in the other's thrall. We both would be totally dependent on other people; we could have great power over others' feelings but no power over our own.

If I have such a belief, when I experience "unpleasant" feelings (sadness, anger, fear…), I can think of myself as a "victim" of others and so can accuse and blame them for that reason ("It's their fault if I'm sad/angry/scared…"); vice versa, when I experience "pleasant" feelings (joy, happiness, gladness…), I can reward others for that reason ("Thanks to him/her, I feel happy…").

Moreover, I feel I bear responsibility (i.e., blame or credit) for the feelings I arouse in other people. In any case, we have always to do with an emotional dependence: my feelings depend on other people (it is they who can make me feel bad or good) and other people's feelings depend on me (it is I who can make them feel good or bad).

[6] The psychotherapeutic point of view: Focus on B

As touched upon in the Introduction, in the psychotherapy field, some theories (such as E. Berne's (1961, 1964, 1972) Transactional Analysis, R. and M. Goulding's Re-Decision Therapy (1978, 1979), F. Perls' (1951) Gestalt therapy, R. Bandler and J. Grinder's (1975) Neuro-Linguistic Programming) maintain a viewpoint which is centred on B's emotional autonomy and independence and which is then antithetical to any that would take A as its focus. According to such theories, no one is responsible for other people's actions, thoughts and feelings; each person is responsible not only for his/her own actions but also for his/her own thoughts and feelings (but not for those of other people); s/he has enough power and capability to be the master of his/her own life. Personal responsibility, power and capability are often denied for different reasons by using, for example, sentences like *You make me feel angry*, so that people consider out of their control feelings which are their own responsibility:

"Sentences of this type, in fact, identify situations in which one person does some act and a second person *responds* by feeling a certain way. The point here is that, although the two events occur one after the other, there is no necessary connection between the act of one person and the response of the other. Therefore, sentences of this type identify a model in which the clients assign responsibility for his emotions to people or forces outside his control. The act itself does not cause the emotion; rather, the emotion is a response generated from a model in which the client takes no responsibility for experiences which he *could* control" (Bandler and Grinder 1975, 51-52).

According to this point of view, in our examples it is not A who, by saying what s/he says, amuses or bores B or makes him/her angry, but, on the contrary, it is B who amuses or bores himself/herself or makes himself/herself angry. In these expressions, verbs and verbal expressions are used in a reflexive way: the grammatical subject and direct object are no longer two different persons (as in the case of *"You* make *me* feel angry"), they are the same and only one person ("*I* make *myself* feel angry").

For that reason, in a psychotherapy session, addressing a client who says "A's talk makes me feel angry", R. and M. Goulding (1978, 1979) do not ask him/her questions such as "What did A tell you to make you feel angry?", because such questions would confirm the client's belief that his/her anger is caused by A. On the contrary, they ask him/her: "When you are listening to A, what do you tell yourself in your head to make yourself angry?". By this kind of questioning, they shift the focus away from A (where it lays in the client's description) to the client himself/herself and they re-propose to him/her his/her anger as a feeling which is totally his/hers, which is dependent on him/her and not on A, as a feeling, then, which s/he can begin to feel himself/herself the master of and be responsible for.

Thus, instead of using sentences with focused-on-A causal expressions such as "A's talk makes me feel angry", it would be more proper to use such *correlative sentences* as "A talks such and such *and* I feel angry / I make myself angry" or *"When* A talks such and such, I feel angry / I make myself angry", i.e., *coordinate* or *subordinate* sentences, in which causative verbs are used reflexively[28].

According to T. Kahler (1978, 277), in fact, the existence of a high correlation between two events (What *you* say and the anger *I* feel) and the probability of predicting exactly that if the first event occurs (i.e., if you say such and such), then the second one will occur too (i.e., I will feel angry), do not necessarily

---

[28] See Claude Steiner's (1977; 2003[2]:79-88) technique called the Action/Feeling Statement.

imply that the former causes the latter. Correlation and probability may have nothing to do, as in the present case, with cause and effect. I can make myself angry whenever you tell me such and such, but that does not mean that you make me feel angry; it only means that, by saying what you say, *you invite me* to feel angry. And invitations may be either accepted or refused....

[7] The Gestalt theoretical point of view: Focus on the relation between A and B

In the field of visual perception, Gestalt psychologist W. Metzger (2001) distinguishes three types of global qualities of the objects we perceive: shape qualities ("round", "linear", ...), material qualities ("smooth", "transparent",...) and expressive qualities ("cheerful", "sad",...). To these he adds a fourth type of qualities, the *Anmutungsweisen* ('modes of appeal': "attractive", "pleasant", "repugnant", "amusing", "boring", interesting",..., see the adjectives in sentences of type 3 in section 2) which, unlike shape, material and expressive qualities, are not *object* qualities, but *relational* qualities: they do not belong to objects as such; they also involve the subject who perceives, since they result with phenomenal immediacy from the *way of being* (*Wesen*) of the perceived object (=A) *in relation to* the *way of being* of the perceiving subject (=B); more precisely, they refer to the particular *effect* (*Wirkung*) that the *relation* between A and B has on B:

"In the case of perceptual Gestalten - and only in the case of such Gestalten - as states of affairs whose nature includes being there for a subject, we distinguish yet another group of properties that are a direct outflow of their essence in its relation to the essence of the subject addressed, but logically must be sharply distinguished from the actual properties of essence, even if in individual cases there may be doubts about the attribution. These are properties such as attractive, repulsive, delightful, disgusting, pleasing, uplifting, depressing, reviving, exciting, soothing, pleasing, boring, encouraging, interesting, offensive, terrible, frightening, frightful, encouraging, appetizing, and so on. This fourth group of qualities, which now really affects the already mentioned relationship between the object of perception and the perceiver - and more precisely its peculiar effect on the latter - is what we call the *Anmutungsweisen (appeal qualities)*." (Translation from Metzger 2001, 64-65)

Metzger's point of view is centred neither only on A nor only on B, but on *both*, or – more precisely – on the *relation* between them. It means that A and B are considered to be on the same level, in that both are 'variables' that contribute to the final result, i.e., the specific *relation* (of attraction, repulsion, etc.)

between A and B, both are 'conditions' of the global effect, the *Anmutungswei-sen*.[29]

Moreover, the *Anmutungsweisen* (qualities of appeal) are Gestalt qualities and, as such, they depend on the *structure* of the phenomenon itself and the structure is given by the roles or functions that its parts play in it and by the mutual relations among parts and whole. In this sense, the *conditions* of the phenomenal existence of the *Anmutungsweisen* are *structural*.

Applied to linguistic communication, where A is not an object but a speaking person, this means that at least two more variables must be added, i.e., what A *says* and the *interpersonal* relation between A and B. Thus, we can say that the *structural conditions*, on which the *Anmutungsweisen* depend, refer to the *dynamic interdependence* of the *phenomenal* features of A, of B, of what A says and of the interpersonal relation between A and B. '*Phenomenal*' means that the structural conditions refer to the dynamic interdependence of *the way in which B 'lives', experiences* A, him/herself, what A says and his/her interpersonal relation with A, in the *momentary* situation (*here and now*) in which communication occurs.

As seen in sections 3 and 4, the common-sense viewpoint tends to consider B's features to be non-existent and to exalt A's and his/her words' features. According to the naïve idea of causality, one cause, A (whether an object or a verbal or non-verbal action of a person) produces one effect, a feeling, in B.[30]

In contrast, Metzger's viewpoint (and more in general, Gestalt theory) argues that the effect of an action by which A "causes" a feeling in B depends not only on the features of the one who "performs the action" (i.e. A), but also on the features of the one who "undergoes the action" (i.e. B). Instead of *cause and effect*, Gestalt theory speaks of *structural conditions*: they do give rise to the 'birth' (phenomenal appearance), 'life'(phenomenal permanence) and 'death' (phenomenal disappearance) of a phenomenon, in our case a feeling.

---

[29] In this respect (A's and B's features are complementary, correlative) Metzger's notion of ‚Anmutungsweisen' is close to the concept of ‚Aufforderungscharakter' or valence introduced by Lewin (1926b).

[30] Cf. Metzger: "[…] the belief in the possibility of a complete knowledge and controllability of the causes of another person's behavior would only be justified if these were to be sought entirely outside the person in question. Here, a concept of cause is more or less tacitly presupposed, which is frequently found in everyday thinking [...]: According to this, the success of an effect would be determined exclusively by the acting object or agent and would be independent of the nature of the object that suffers the effect." (Translated from Metzger 2001[6], 247).

Lewin (1936, 213) defines *systematic causation* in the following way: "An event is considered as a function of the total situation at a particular time. The cause of an event is always the interrelation between several facts".

In terms of his *psychological field* or *psychological life space* theory this means that "to understand or predict the psychological behaviour (*B*) one has to determine for every kind of psychological event (actions, emotions, expressions, etc.) the momentary whole situation, that is, the momentary structure and the state of the person (*P*) and of the psychological environment (*E*). $B = f (PE)$. Every fact that exists psychobiologically must have a position in this field and only facts that have such position have dynamic effects (are causes of events)."[31]

[8] Wesenseigenschaften (expressive qualities; „tertiary qualities") vs Anmutungsweisen (appeal qualities)

Though the *Anmutungsweisen* result from B's relation with A and refer to the effect that such a relation has on B's feelings, everyday linguistic communication attributes such qualities not to B but to A.

When I say, for example, "That movie is amusing", "This exercise is boring" or "Mary is depressing", I use the adjectives "amusing", "boring" and "depressing" as if they were object qualities, in particular as if they were *expressive qualities* [Wesenseigenschaften; "tertiary qualities"] of the movie, of the exercise, of Mary, as when I say, "That movie is cheerful" or "Mary is sad". Expressive qualities such as "cheerful" and "sad", which are the movie's and Mary's properties, have to be distinguished from *Anmutungsweisen* such as "amusing" and "depressing", which refer to the effect that my relation with the movie or with Mary has on *my* feelings.

A movie may be cheerful and not amuse me, just as my interaction with a sad person may not depress me. Cheerfulness and sadness are the movie's and Mary's properties, they do not depend on my feelings; in contrast, amusement and depression are feelings which *I* experience over the movie and Mary. A person other than me could experience different feelings. But, instead of saying, as it would be more correct, "I feel depressed, when I'm with Mary" (because, for example, she is sad), language allows me to say "Mary is depressing me" or even simply "Mary is depressing".

---

[31] On the relational character of causal facts see Lewin 1935, Chapter II; Lewin 1936, Chapter V. On the philosophical and psychological problem of causality and the Gestalt theoretical approach to it see Michotte 1963, Chapter I and XVII, and Bozzi 1969, Chapter V and VI. On the pre-scientific concept of 'cause' and the scientific notion of 'conditions' see also Metzger 2001, Chapter VII.

In this way, qualities which are *relative to the perceiving subject* are presented by language as *object's absolute qualities* and the relation between object and subject is presented as a cause-effect relation: "I" - who am the experiential or phenomenal subject that feels depressed, amused or bored - become a linguistic or grammatical object, a "me", i. e. a direct object of the action of something else (movie, exercise) or someone else (Mary) which in its (or her) turn becomes the subject of the sentence: "It's the movie that amuses me", "It's the exercise that bores me", "It's Mary who depresses me". Again a causal structure appears focused on the other-than-I, whether object or person. Yet, if the feelings I experience over objects and persons depend on me too, how is it possible to maintain that it is the other-than-I which causes my feelings and to say "That movie is amusing me", "This exercise is boring me", "Mary is depressing me", "You make me feel angry", i.e. how is it possible to use a linguistic structure according to which my feelings depend on objects and on other persons?

We could then ask ourselves: why in everyday usage is causal language focused on A? How did a syntactic-semantic and conceptual organization focused on A come to prevail over other possible ones?

[9] Why is causal language focused on A? Three possible answers

9.1 *The common-sense answer*

The common-sense answer takes the following line: we talk the way we do, i.e., we use causal sentences of type 1-3, because feeling-causality *really exists; it is true* that others make us feel a certain way, and just as true that we make others feel a certain way.

If we apply Gestalt theory, in particular Metzger's *critical realism* approach, to the relationships between language and the non-linguistic reality which language refers to, such an answer would be thought of as "naïve", because it implies that language refers to *transphenomenal reality*: here the existence of causal expressions in language is accounted for by the existence of affective causality in transphenomenal reality.

In contrast, according to the "critical" viewpoint of Gestalt theory, language refers to *phenomenal reality*, i.e., not to the *world* (transphenomenal reality) but to our *experience of the world* (phenomenal reality) (Michotte 1959; Zuczkowski 1995; 2003; 2005; 2006; Zuczkowski, Riccioni 2010; Zuczkowski, Bongelli, Riccioni 2017). Thus, the answer to our question has to be looked for, first of all, within the scope of the relations between language and phenomenal reality.

9.2 *The linguistic determinism answer*

If in our consideration of the relations between language and phenomenal reality we take up the hypothesis that the syntactic and semantic structures of language determine in native speakers a particular *conceptualization* of their experience, a specific *cognitive organization* of reality (see, for example, Whorf 1956), then the following answer becomes possible: we believe, we think, we are convinced that other people cause our feelings and vice versa because our language gives us a particular 'structure of thought' which conveys precisely that causal logic. In short, we *think* of emotional causality the way we do because we *talk* the way we do.

Metzger (2001) thinks of phenomenal reality as a *continuum* in which it is possible to distinguish *Encountered phenomenal reality* (here and now I perceive/see/hear… something) from *Represented phenomenal reality* (here and now I think/believe/imagine/remember…something). According to this view, the linguistic determinism answer, compared with the common-sense answer, would have the merit of considering not transphenomenal reality but thought (i.e., Represented phenomenal reality) to be the referent of language.

But such an answer seems to be only a pseudo-explanation, for it does not answer our question, it simply shifts the focus of the problem elsewhere: indeed, we think that way because we talk that way, but *why do we talk that way*? Where does that way of talking come from?

9.3 *A Gestalt specific answer*

A Gestalt specific answer to our question comes from Albert Michotte's (1881-1965) experimental phenomenology of perception of causality. His experiments show that (1) causality is a phenomenal datum, (2) it is a perceptual (= Encountered) phenomenal datum before being or becoming a Represented phenomenal datum, and (3) it is a perceptual phenomenal datum without a transphenomenal correlate.

The word "causality" is used by Michotte (1954/1963, 1962) in the most common sense of the term: the physical action of one thing over another, the production of an event by another, as for example the action of one billiard-ball that hits another. The problem that interests Michotte can be summed up by the following question: can we *see* an object *cause* with its action an *effect* on another object? In other terms, can we have a direct, immediate visual experience of causality? Just to remain in the example, can we see one billiard-ball *strike* another, i.e., *cause* its movement?

The European psychology which was dominant till the beginning of the twentieth century believed that we could see only what has correspondence in the field of stimuli (psychophysical constancy hypothesis).

It is well known that in physical causality there is no 'local' (=point) stimulus which corresponds to the causal link, i.e., to the 'influence' that for instance the push of an object exerts on the movement of another object; therefore, there can be no perception of causality. Perception would limit itself to the movements of the two objects, one after the other. The causal link would be added to the visual data by the cognitive systems (thought, memory, etc.), for instance by an 'interpretation' of the visual data based on past experience and acquired knowledge.

The point of view of the scientific psychology found wide support in the philosophical tradition, particularly in David Hume: in the famous example of the billiard, indeed, he argues that we can perceive only the movements of the balls, not the causal link that joins them together. Perception limits itself to movements and time relations of simultaneity and succession. The notion of causality results, according to Hume, from the regularity of movements' succession and from their repetition, which leads to make associations, habits, according to which, in the presence of the antecedent, we expect the consequent, i. e. the appearance of this latter when the former occurs.

According to Michotte, this kind of theory is no longer tenable since when Gestalt psychologists highlighted that the combinations of stimuli produce on the perceptual level some global impressions which are very different from the sum of the impressions that the stimuli produce when they act in isolation, separately. Furthermore, specific perceptual data, as Max Wertheimer's experiments on stroboscopic movement show, do not correspond to any local stimulation. Gestalt psychologists' experiments have shown that perceptual phenomena are not due, in principle, to past experience and acquired knowledge; on the contrary, they are *primitive, original* phenomena, i. e. they are the direct response of the perceptual system to a whole of stimulations that impose a specific organization of the perceptual field.

If so, then the problem of the perception of causality can be put in a new way and experimentally verified: are we still sure that it is impossible *to see* one physical or mechanical event causing another and that only their succession can be perceived?

In his principal book on this topic, Michotte (1954/1963) presents about one hundred experiments that nowadays can be re-made on the screen of a computer.[32] To our purposes, it is enough to recall only the *launching effect* (*l'effet lancement*) and its component parts, the *approaching* and *departing effects* (*les effets rapprochement et écartement*).

Experiment 1: the approaching effect

On a white screen the experimental subjects (Ss) see two stationary little squares, one black to the left (A) and another red in the middle (B). At a given moment, A starts moving towards B at moderate speed and it stops when it

---

[32] For an English translation of the main French papers written by Michotte and comments on his experimental work see Thinès, Costall, Butterworth 1991.

gets in touch with B. Ss usually say to see that A approaches B, goes near B, joins B, and the like; they have no causal impression, i.e., no impression that A's movement *tends to continue and is obstructed* by B nor that B *exerts any attraction on* A. A's movement is perceived as A's own movement, i.e., *autonomous* (= it appears to belong to A) and *spontaneous* (= it does not appear to be caused by B).

Experiment 2: the departing effect

To another group of Ss the experimenter shows the final configuration of experiment 1: A and B are contiguous and stationary in the middle of the screen. At a given moment, B moves towards the right side of the screen, while A remains stationary. Some Ss say they see the right and red half of a two-coloured rectangle detaching itself from the other black half and going away. Other Ss say they see two stationary and adjacent squares, the right red one then moves away and leaves the other. B's movement, as A's movement in experiment 1, is perceived as autonomous and spontaneous. Also, in this experiment Ss have no impression of causality, i.e., for instance a *rejection* of A by B.

Experiment 3: the launching effect

Experiments 1 and 2 are joined together in order to obtain one single experiment. If the 'psychophysical constancy hypothesis' were true, we should expect a succession of the two impressions of approaching and departing.

Ceteris paribus, as long as the temporal interval between the arrival of A near B and the departure of B from A remains sufficiently wide, Ss' reports do not differ from those given in experiments 1 and 2: they say they see, for example, that "A goes near B *and then* B goes away from A". These two sentences are co-ordinated by the conjunction *and* plus the temporal adverb *then* which both mean that Ss see two separate and distinct events following one another, i.e., independent from each other: first the approaching, then the departing effect.

On the other hand, when the temporal interval between 1 and 2 is sufficiently short, the impression is completely different and new: Ss see an *action* by A over B; they say to see that "A hits, strikes B, gives it a push, launches B forward". Though there is no local stimulus that corresponds to the influence that A exerts on B, the causal impression is clear-cut: it is A's push that makes B depart, that produces its movement.

This experiment shows that the launching effect is not a simple juxtaposition of the approaching and departing effects; it is something more and different: Ss say to see one single event of causal type, one single *action*: A launches B. A is the agent, it is A that makes everything: it moves and displaces B. A's movement keeps on appearing autonomous and spontaneous. On the contrary, B's movement is no longer perceived as spontaneous and autonomous, but as *caused* by A. At the physical level, i.e. at the level of the stimulation system, there is no difference between A's and B's movements in the three experiments; yet, at the phenomenal level, i.e. the level of perception, B's movement in the third experiment loses the phenomenal feature of being autonomous and spontaneous and takes that of being a simple passive *displacement* caused by A.

The launching effect shows that at the phenomenal level we can have an immediate impression of causality, though at the physical level, i.e., at the level of the stimulation system, A's and B's movements are independent from each other, i.e., though there is no stimulus that corresponds to A's causal influence over B.

The production of B's movement by A is directly perceived, seen. It is not an inference, or a meaning added to an impression of movement, nor an interpretation based on past experience and acquired knowledge.

The causal impression is a perceptual Gestalt that depends on a precise system of stimulation, i.e., on some specific *structural conditions* of *temporal, spatial and kinetic* type, and on the laws of the perceptual organization. For instance, *if* A's and B's movements follow one another within an optimal time interval (temporal condition), *if* the trajectories of the two movements are contiguous and in the same direction (spatial condition), *if* the relationship between A's and B's speeds remains within optimal limits (kinetic condition), *then* the impression of launch occurs. The conditions are structural since each of them interacts with the others, thus forming a particular system of relationships, i.e., a particular structure. If the experimenter modifies only one of these, the whole structure changes and the impression of launch disappears.

Therefore, the perception of causality is a primitive and *specific* phenomenon that originates in the perceptual field itself, when the required conditions of stimulation are given, independently from acquired experience. This means that causal phenomena have no *extrinsic* meaning (Michotte 1950b, 1955a, 1955b), i.e. a meaning which is learned by experience and attributed, under the influence of acquired knowledge, to single impressions of movements only contiguous in time and space; causal phenomena are not the result of a more or less direct 'interpretation' of the perceptual data. The addition of an acquired meaning would not complete these phenomena at all; any interpretation of the 'data' would be superfluous since it would enrich their content in nothing : these phenomena do not need to be completed in any way, they are already complete, in that they have their meaning in themselves, i.e., their meaning is *intrinsic, immanent* (Michotte 1950b, 1955a, 1955b) in what one perceives *hic et nunc*, they are full of sense in themselves.

Thus, the answer to our initial question (why in everyday talk causal structures are centred exclusively on A?) could be found by seeing the perceptual experience which language refers to as governing: the correlate of the language of feeling-causality would lie, first of all, on the perceptual phenomenal level.

If I am convinced (i.e. if I do not doubt it) that other people cause my feelings, it is because I find the highest degree of consistency between what I *experience* daily in the course of my communication with others and the meaning that these particular causal expressions offer me in conceptualizing my *experience*. Here the word "experience" has to be understood not as "Represented phenomenal reality" but as "Encountered phenomenal reality" since the causal link between language and feelings is first of all not a representation, a thought, but a perception, and only afterwards does that link become a representation (thought, belief, conviction or prejudice).

In line with Michotte, we claim that affective causality is a *perceptual* (Encountered) phenomenal datum *in absence of a transphenomenal correlate*. In brief, affective causality is as apparent as the mechanical causality studied by Michotte or the stroboscopic movement by Wertheimer.

10. Feeling-causality in linguistic communication and the 'tool' effect

If we wanted to draw a specific analogy between Michotte's experiments and affective causality in the linguistic communication, the two squares A and B would not be enough, since in the communicative situation there is a third variable that can be perceived also by an outer observer (as the experimental subject is), i.e., what A says; we thus need a third square referring to A's words. Indeed, as seen in section 3, A makes B feel angry *by* saying what s/he says. Therefore, A's words are a *means*, an *instrument* in order for A to cause effects in B.

If so, we think that the experiment, among the numerous ones made by Michotte, which could allow us to draw a specific analogy with the linguistic communication is 'the tool effect'(Michotte 1951).

On the screen, halfway between A and B, Ss see a third square, C. At a given moment, A moves towards C and, as soon as A stops near C, C moves towards B and, as soon as C stops near B, B moves away.

Ss have no impression of two successive launchings (A launches C and C launches B), but rather of a single global action: A launches B through the intermediation of C, i.e., A immediately appears as the only one responsible for the launch of B, or, more precisely, for the impact C-B which launches B. It is A "which does everything" and is the sole agent. C's movement is neither spontaneous nor autonomous, is passive: it is not C that launches B through its own power; C simply serves to transfer the blow, that it received by A, to B. C is thus the mere agent of transmission of the blow given by A. *The intervention of the intermediary object C appears to be integrated as a constituent part with the action of the motor object A; it is this which gives C the characteristic phenomenal aspect of a 'tool'.*

In everyday life, the hammer manipulated by the user is an example of what gives us a direct impression of being an intermediary, that is a means of execution, which is itself devoid of any initiative. We attribute quite different roles to the respective effects of the initial mover and the intermediary: the latter is essentially subordinated to the former, the tool is only the means of performing the action of the user. Analogous are the roles that in the communicative situation we attribute to A (the initial mover, the speaker) and to his/her words (the intermediate C) which both cause B's movement, i.e. the listener's anger (or whatever).

11. Emotions, movements, causality

As far as emotions and causality are concerned, according to Michotte it is interesting to take into consideration those data which

"are summed up in the statement, made time and time again by writers concerned with introspective psychology, that emotions, needs, and tendencies are directly linked with the events which give rise to them, or with other events which result from them, Here there is not just a simple succession of independent phenomena, but an *intrinsic* bond which observers, rightly or wrongly, often describe in terms suggesting a causal connexion." (Michotte 1963,14)

Thus, the problem of the perception of mechanical causality can be put in relation with the problem concerning

"the link between emotions and the events which seem to produce their appearance. The part played by such events is often described in language implying the presence of causality." (Michotte 1963, 282)

In addition, however,

"the present approach supplies a methodological pointer, since it raises the question of whether the study of emotion could be helped by knowledge obtained in connexion with the perception of kinematic functional relations.

This approach seems all the more justified since there are very marked similarities, as has often been pointed out, between emotions and movements. This is exemplified by some of our habitual ways of talking, and in particular by our very use of the word 'emotion', i.e. 'movement of the soul'. Besides this there are countless familiar idioms, e.g. 'I was *struck* all of a heap', 'It *shook* me to pieces', "I was *overwhelmed* by grief", 'I was *transported* with joy', 'I am deeply *impressed*', 'It *pierced* me to the quick', 'It *crushed* me', 'It *got me down*', 'It *knocked me flat*', 'I. am *bursting* with enthusiasm', 'I feel *drawn* towards', "That is *repulsive*', 'I am *stricken* with grief, 'That is *attractive*', "That gave me a *shock*', and many others. All these terms not only have a kinematic significance in addition they clearly imply *mechanical action*. They thus indicate once again the important part played by kinaesthetic impressions in this field, and they are evidence that the emotions have a motor character more or Jess similar to that which appears in obvious cases of mechanical causality, especially of the propulsion type. This does not mean, of course, that this motor aspect completely exhausts the whole phenomenal character of emotion." (Michotte 1963, 283)

Therefore, emotions can now

"rightly be regarded as *functional relations*, just like all the relations which we have so far considered, such as launching, entraining, approach, withdrawal, pursuit, passing over, overtaking, compressing, traction, transport, etc. Like these, emotions are *changes in an object (wiz. the self)* **apparently** *occurring as a function of another object*, and they arise in a large number of qualitatively different forms." (Michotte 1963, 282)

"It should be made clear immediately, however, that this problem has nothing to do with the 'objective' conditions in which emotions are aroused; the issue is **purely a phenomenal one**. When an emotional state develops under the influence of factors whose nature we need not consider for the moment, this emotional state usually has the **appearance** of being intrinsically linked with a definite phenomenon, and it is *this phenomenon* which produces fear, pleasure, or pain, provokes disgust, or arouses bad temper or anger. We need therefore to examine whether on these occasions there are genuine *causal* **impressions** and why they appear in such circumstances." (Michotte 1963, 282)

As in the case of mechanical causality, also in that of affective causality the study of the *phenomenal conditions* of the origin, permanence and disappearance of a particular feeling become fundamental. One of the most suitable contexts where to carry on such a study seems to be the psychotherapeutic one.

12. The place of emotional experience in Gestalt Theoretical Psychotherapy

Gestalt Theoretical Psychotherapy as a psychotherapy method consistently oriented on Gestalt psychology focuses strongly on the human being as a social being and thus as a relational being. In this understanding, this is closely connected with a special interest in the emotional experience of the human being. The rationale for this emerges from the following considerations (see also Stemberger & Sternek 2019):

From the point of view of Gestalt Theoretical Psychotherapy, the emotional experience of a person is a form of particularly prägnant ego-world cognition. In this context, the characteristics of the person and his environment are particularly pronounced, the person-environment relationship has a specific structure, and specifically directed impulses for movement and behavior are inherent in the experience of the ego-world-relationship. Accordingly, the experience of feelings is not an experience limited to or enclosed in the person, even if the person can be experienced as the "bearer" of the feeling; the experience of feelings is always an *experience of* the ego-world-relationship - the characteristics associated with it are never only those of the person, but always also those of the world: a person who is happy also "has" a "joy-world" with specific structural and essential characteristics and a specific dynamic, a person who is angry also has a "world of anger" with the characteristic features of it.

Corresponding to the existential conditions of life of man, other people and such facts are particularly emphasized in his ego-world experience, which refer to the co-human living together. This also applies to his emotional experience: In the given situation the essence of one's own person and that of the other person is concisely given, as well as the essence of the relationship between the two in a characteristically shaped world and also the dynamics laid down in this situation as a movement-impulse or movement-"order" of the two persons in this world - away from each other or towards each other, etc.

In this specific ego-world experience, certain causal connections are not always phenomenally given, but especially in interpersonal situations they are quite often. It is true that there are also situations where, for example, a person in happy company suddenly becomes sad and the reasons for this sudden change are puzzling to him, at least for the time being. But there are also situations in which it is already more or less clearly given in the experience itself how these feelings have come about. The phenomena whose backgrounds were treated in the preceding sections often appear here: The other person and what this person says or does or has said or done is experienced as the cause of the feeling just experienced; also certain feeling states perceived in other people are experienced as having been caused by one's own behavior and one's own expressions.

Now people actually do act on each other, even if not in the linear-causal way as the naïve experience in the cases described above suggests. In the physical environment, which is common to them, their physical organisms affect each other (among other things also on the way of sound waves, if something is said and heard), which is reflected by cybernetic regulation processes, mediated by physical and chemical processes also in their brain activity and enters there in the PPN (psychophysical level) in specific way into the stream of the phenomenally experienced.

The interaction between organisms in the macro-physical world and the mutual influence between two experienced persons in the phenomenal world differ essentially. In the phenomenal world the interaction is determined by *field relations*, which is not true for the mutual impact of the respective organisms in the macro-physical world and the "transfer" of this impact to the phenomenal world.. Because of this peculiarity of the phenomenal world, no simple linear-causal causations from A to B take place there either, although processes - as the preceding sections have discussed - can be experienced as such. However, this peculiarity also makes the phenomenal world flexible or plastic in a certain way - by restructuring in the phenomenal world, phenomenally given causation relations can also be loosened or cancelled again and new ones can be formed.

Such processes can also unfold spontaneously in psychotherapeutic processes or as part of volitional changes. Because man wants to understand himself and his life and also needs this understanding existentially in order to find his way in it and to shape it, causal relationships have special significance in his life and experience. This will now be discussed in more detail on the basis of a few selected questions and examples.

13. Manifestations, effects, therapeutic options

In Gestalt Theoretical Psychotherapy we assume that like all phenomenal processes also those of naïve causality of feelings are understandable and have meaning and purpose in the mental life of man. To this end, a few examples will now be analyzed. The point is to work out the conditions under which this naïve feeling-causality occurs and to trace the forces that play a role in it. Naïve emotional causality becomes a therapeutic issue where it restricts or blinds a person or contributes to particular difficulties in life, especially in living together with others. It is then a matter of finding ways of overcoming such naïve emotional causality by removing the ground from it through a restructuring of the psychic field.

Before naïve feeling-causality is clothed in words, it is *experienced*. The phenomenal world is actually ordered at this moment in a way that it is undeniably clear that a certain feeling is caused by another person or that one oneself has caused certain feelings in someone else. Therefore, it is about psychologically real and therefore effective causal connections which nobody can explain away.

The experienced dynamic order, of which these contexts are essential congruents, has far-reaching effects on the entirety of experience and behavior. How this order comes about depends not only on conditions *in the* person's *environment* (e.g., the timely succession of events experienced as causation), but also on conditions in the *person himself* (his need situation and which intentions he is currently pursuing) - it is thus a result of the *overall situation*.

To understand what is meant here, a few examples:

Example 1: A child experiences himself as the cause of his parents' discord and their divorce:

Here, as a rule, a "misunderstanding" is at play, which stems from the opacity of the circumstances in which the child finds itself, insidiously or abruptly. The discord between the parents is an event from which the child experiences itself excluded in a threatening way. Following a well-known analysis by Max

Wertheimer and Heinrich Schulte[33], one can envision the further development as follows: Since the child experiences himself as dependent on his parents, the experience of being separated from them is a frightening, existentially threatening situation. In contrast, a restructuring of this situation, in which the child can experience himself as the cause of parental disruption, is a reordering of the child's world, in which he is still or anew important to the parents and closely connected to them through this causal relationship. This ordering of his world is also agonizing, but it is still easier to bear than not playing any role at all for the parents, not belonging at all and being completely powerless. In this case, the experience of the relationship of causation can be understood dynamically in such a way that it bridges an otherwise unbearable gap to the parents and the whole event and at the same time frees the child somewhat from its powerlessness - if it has caused the rift, it is perhaps also within its power to undo it. Therapeutically, it would then be a matter of looking for other ways in which this belonging can be re-established and experienced.

Example 2: A couple newly in love experiences their feelings of happiness as caused by their partner - he/she makes me happy and I make him/her happy. Therefore, they never want to let go of each other. The thought of possibly losing the other is unbearable.

In this case, too, a "short circuit" is at play: When we are together, we are happy, so the other person must be the cause of this wonderful state of feeling. When he is there, I feel good, when he is not there, I feel bad - so he must be the cause of me feeling good (or bad in his absence). It's not the relationship that makes me happy, it's the other person.

If one remembers the so-called „Gestalt laws" (the Gestalt factors), one thinks here immediately of a "pair formation". „Pair" does not mean the loving couple in this context, but the union of two circumstances because of the factor of the proximity and the common fate (in this case of the simultaneous appearance of the other person and the emotional state). What "inner" conditions can it have that a person - at least for a certain time - experiences the other as the causer of his feeling of happiness and possibly also himself as the causer of the other's feeling of happiness? The preconditions for the naïve feeling-causality here are usually to be sought in the person's striving for togetherness or attachment, which at least temporarily takes on this oversimplified ("primitive-praegnant") form. Only the insight that what makes the person happy is not the other person in itself, but the relationship between the two, to which both also

---

[33] See Heinrich Schulte (1924): Versuch einer Theorie der paranoischen Eigenbeziehung und Wahnbildung. Fully translated into English by Erwin Levy 1986.

contribute and have to contribute, makes more praegnant forms of relationship possible.

Example 3: A young employee can hardly stand the presence of his superior - even if the latter says nothing at all to him, "he always gives him the feeling of being completely incapable".

Here, too, we are dealing with an oversimplified and thus distorted world of the person concerned. It is radically simplified to an incomprehensible - almost magical - but all the more effective state of causation of feelings by the boss. A closer look will perhaps show that there may be certain connecting factors in the nature and physiognomy of the boss, perhaps also connected with similarities to earlier authority figures in the life of the person concerned, which make one think of "transference phenomena". However, this does not answer the question, neither for the current nor for earlier situations, on the basis of which "inner" dynamics of the person concerned and his relationship to his environment these circumstances can become effective and bring about and maintain just this oversimplified order of his world. The only thing that seems clear is that at the given time this order, distorted by simplification, is preferred to a more differentiated one, which may seem all too threatening to the self-esteem of the person concerned. Overcoming such a distorting simplified order requires a self-critical examination of one's own attitudes of entitlement, one's own abilities and the perceived demands of the job instead of a simple centering on the "boss's judgment" and perhaps all too naïve ideas and wishes regarding one's own professional life.

Example 4: A psychotherapist repeatedly feels strongly unsettled by a certain client, something he otherwise hardly knows about himself.

The same considerations would now have to be made as in the third example just discussed. It is mentioned here to counteract a misunderstanding that naïve emotional causality in psychotherapy would only be effective with the clients.

Therapists as well as their clients experience dynamic orders of their phenomenal world inside and outside of therapy, which usually withstand a "reality check", but sometimes may turn out to be erroneous. Causation relations are a variety of such orders. They take on a weighty role already because it often has tangible consequences for one's own experience and behavior how one experiences the coming into being of certain facts and states.

If I feel a draft in the room and assume that the cause is that two windows are open, the "reality check" is that I close the two windows (or at least one) and the draft then stops. In fact, however, already in this case the causality relations are not so simple - the opened windows are a boundary condition for the draught, but not its cause (air pressure and temperature differences). In everyday life, however, in such a case this kind of "reality check" and its result are usually sufficient for us.

However, as the above examples have at least indicated, life does not always let us get away with such simple explanations and solutions. If the difficulties involved lead into psychotherapy or become visible there in connection with other problems, it will ultimately be a matter of "restructuring the field" (Canestrari & Trombini 1975, 2019; Galli & Trombini 2013), resulting in a more differentiated and yet, against all previous fears, well livable reorganization of one's world.[34]

---

[34] For such a restructuring, it can also be helpful in practice to try other formulations and to pay attention to what a world would look like to which these other formulations would fit. Instead of "You're making me angry," you might try, "You say that and I realize I'm getting angry. How come?" For reasons of space, the interrelations between what is said and what is experienced cannot be explored further here - their treatment is reserved for a separate article.

7. The Task of Diagnostics in Gestalt Theoretical Psychotherapy

Doris Beneder & Bernadette Lindorfer

The understanding of mental health and illness in Gestalt Theoretical Psychotherapy (GTP) assumes that people's behavioral and experiential patterns regarded as mental disorders arise from attempts to cope with the challenges of life, especially in the interpersonal sphere. They follow the same regularities of dynamic order as the ones considered normal and healthy. This understanding also corresponds to the conception of the task of diagnostics in Gestalt Theoretical Psychotherapy.

Diagnosis and therapy: not *two* processes, but *one*. The client as diagnostician

Whatever happens in therapy can reveal something of the psychological situation of the person concerned and of the *inherent and effective forces and possibilities*. In this respect, every therapeutic step also carries a diagnostic potential, and vice versa, every diagnostic step a therapeutic one. Every new diagnostic insight is in itself already a change in the therapeutic process and can thus become the starting point for further changes, which in turn lead to new diagnostic perspectives. From this perspective it follows inevitably that in GTP psychotherapeutic diagnosis is not seen as a separate or upstream component of therapy, but as an inherent part of psychotherapeutic work.

GTP relies on the interplay of two types of diagnosis: on the one hand, on the diagnostic process, findings, and assumptions on the part of the *therapist*, and on the other hand, on the diagnostic process and the diagnosis on the part of the *clients*. By the client's diagnosis, it is not meant that the clients themselves adopt one of the classifications of mental disorders from ICD or DSM, but that they come to a clear assessment of their situations including their own persons, the requirements of their lives and their possibilities and resources. The path to this goal of clarification is the diagnostic process, which the therapist cannot spare the client, but in which the therapist can accompany the clients both professionally and with human compassion. Ultimately, this diagnostic process and the diagnosis on the part of the clients are crucial for the therapeutic success. It is the *clients* who must become clear about themselves, their situations, and the possible and necessary steps of change. This is the subject of the process of the clients' self-diagnosis in the course of the therapy and at the same time an essential and decisive part of the therapy.

Accordingly, the diagnostic task on the part of the therapist consists of nothing else than the professional and human-solidary guidance and support of the client in this process. The fact that the therapists can phrase their understanding and assessment of the client's situation in terms, constructs and categorizations, which go beyond the common everyday language dialogue with the client, e.g., for the exchange with the therapist's professional environment, does not interfere with the priority given to the client's self-diagnosis.

The object of psychotherapeutic diagnostics is - theoretically expressed – the "persons in their current situations", i.e., in their life spaces, which also includes their currently experienced environments. As a holistic theory, Gestalt theory assumes a continuum of events whose units result from segregations within the field (cf. Rausch 1952 cited in Galli 2005, 14). The life space includes in certain constellations more the dynamic conditions of the *momentary* situation, in others more those of the *life* situation. Already in the initial session of the therapy the joint exploration of the currently effective psychological situation of the client primarily follows the ways of the client and not a prefabricated system and structuring, for example in the sense of a systematic anamnesis. Here, the "top-down" approach applies as well– it is not about a systematic collection of details, but about an approach to the dynamic character of the client's situation. The focus of attention is on the clients' goals in their current situations and in life, as expressed in this dynamic, and on their interpersonal relationships, with which the pursuit and achievement of these goals are usually intimately linked.

Diagnostics and respect

When the therapists as diagnosticians make statements about the psychological situation of their clients, in the end they always speak about their own experience of the client and not at all about "how the client *is*". As the Italian Gestalt psychologist Giuseppe Galli explains in detail, Gestalt theory can be called a "school of respect" – in contrast, for example, to the "schools of suspicion". This is also crucial for its diagnostic ideas. Especially for the diagnostic side of the psychotherapeutic process, one can quickly adopt an arrogant attitude, which Galli describes as follows: "The psychological opposites to respect are intrusiveness and the possessiveness of knowing everything about the other and thus 'owning' him." (Galli 2017, 4). It would be a completely false claim to believe that one's own expertise can quickly provide a clear view ("see-through"?) of the deep layers of the other person's personality and psychological situation. Psychotherapeutic diagnosis is rather a process of gradual opening up between the persons involved, of mutual understanding and being understood, adapted at any moment to the client's working speed. An approach "from the outside" as an expert who imposes a judgment on the other person in the sense of a diagnostic label does not fit the Gestalt theoretical perspective.

Besides a respectful attitude towards ourselves, the client and the therapeutic setting, the critical-realistic perspective of Gestalt theory has another consequence, namely that therapist and client are "dependent" on each other in a mutual process. In this process, the therapists place their own experience, as it were, as a diagnostic tool at the service of the client and the common therapeutic task: The natural *factual* focus of the therapeutic situation is on the clarification of the client's situation and lifeworld. The focus of the therapist's *attention*, however, can change again and again in the course of a session and also draw on her own experience. Thus, the focus of attention can shift to the therapist's own reactions to the client or also to the relationship between the therapist and the client as experienced by the therapist in a specific way at the given moment (cf. Stemberger 2013). Therefore, important diagnostic conclusions can also be drawn again and again, which can flow into the exchange with the client and finally also contribute to different therapeutic strategies and interventions.

The attitude and approach to the therapeutic relationship are also derived from the critical-realistic stance (see Sternek in the current volume). The ideal type is the idea of an approximately coordinative therapeutic relationship, whereby the factual focus is naturally on the needs and difficulties, but also on the possibilities of the client. As a rule, clients cannot meet their therapists in such an autonomous way from the very beginning; rather, it is important to establish the framework from the very beginning in such a way that this becomes increasingly possible. Galli (2005) describes some concise (prägnant) forms of „social virtues ", which are part of the therapist's tasks to develop and maintain, so that the therapeutic situation can become a situation of "creative freedom" (Metzger 1962/2022). The virtues that characterize the therapeutic relationship include devotion, gratitude, wonder, repentance, trust and sincerity. Especially the analysis of the psychological contrasts of these attitudes proves to be a source of inspiration for describing and understanding the therapeutic relationship, its possibilities and pitfalls.

The positive effect of sincere trust in the client's inner forces has an immediate impact when the client comes to the therapy session in a situation of misery and hopelessness, and when towards the end at least a little confidence and hope has arisen that can carry the process further.

Insight into one's own situation and its demands is usually not enough to overcome a crisis. It also requires encouragement, confidence and empowerment, and not only the discovery of one's own strengths and possibilities, but also those of one's fellow human beings – and then the decision to tackle what is necessary.

Do not look for diseases, but understand the psychological situation

"If the relationship between therapist and client is sustainable, then the client will want the therapist not only to accompany him/her through her phenomenal world in a friendly way, but in a knowledgeable and, in the best sense, factual way, not only by looking, but also in the ensuing next steps of working on necessary changes. The client will hope, at least at times, that the therapist will have good ideas about how best to proceed in clarifying the situation" (Stemberger 2016, 34).

In GTP we try to meet these justified expectations - technically speaking – with the methodical approach of force field analysis, which we have taken over from Kurt Lewin and adapted for the field of psychotherapy. The aim is to make the dynamic constellations of conditions of the forces currently at work in the client's life space tangible and to trace the laws that are effective in them, from which conclusions can then be drawn about the therapeutic possibilities for action, the method to be chosen and the prognosis.

The focus of interest is the currently effective own and foreign will goals and the obstacles that stand in the way of their pursuit. Information about this is often given by the emotional experience, with which the person in a concise manner grasps the dynamics of his or her momentary situation. In general, force field analysis prefers to use "experimental variation" of the various circumstances of the situation, true to the motto attributed to Kurt Lewin: "If you want to understand something, try to change it." This is done by means of conversation, play, various creative outlets, and any other variation.

Stemberger (2010) illustrates such a procedure with the example of a client with depressive symptoms, whose life situation was recorded and understood as one of „decision avoidance ". In doing so, the claim to develop a general theory of depression does not arise, because only concrete things can have an effect and only through the analysis of the concrete individual case can dynamics become visible. Such a situation-centered approach can theoretically and empirically be based on a wealth of elaborations and investigations, especially in the tradition of the Lewin School. As classic examples of the analysis of psychological situations, we may mention the study of the psychological situation in reward and punishment and the entire Berlin experiments on the psychology of action and affect (Lewin1931; De Rivera 1976; review article on the psychological situation: Stemberger 2021b). These are examples of how, by grasping the dynamic constellations, one can arrive at an understanding of the symptoms, barriers, and possibilities that currently determine a person's situation.

"Correct grasping of what 'is' is not only an 'explanation' of what happens, but at the same time also a signpost for what *can and should happen.*" (Stemberger 2010a, 345, referring to Kurt Lewin)

Again and again, the course of therapy will also be the subject of diagnostic reflection. On the one hand, of course, this applies to the clients, who will repeatedly ask themselves where they stand in the course of the therapy, whether they have come closer to their goals and what road still lies ahead of them. On the other hand, the diagnosis of the course of therapy is also a topic for the therapist – is the therapy progressing, in what way is this noticeable, is it already coming to a conclusion? In the current volume, suggestions based on Gestalt theory can be found in the contribution by Trombini, Trombini & Stemberger.

Relationship to the classificatory systems of ICD and DSM

Methodologically, the diagnostic procedure in GTP is thus oriented towards the phenomenological-experimental procedure of the change-activating force field or life space analysis according to Kurt Lewin, taking into account the "six characteristics of work on the living" according to Wolfgang Metzger (cf. Böhm in the current volume). The relationship to the classification systems ICD and DSM, which are alien to psychotherapy, is thereby critical with regard to their meta-theoretical position and orientation, and at the same time pragmatic with regard to the need for psychotherapists to familiarize themselves with them in order to be able to engage in exchange (or: interact) with other health professions and institutions. Furthermore, the need is seen for therapist and client to deal with the effects of such classifications on experience and behavior on the part of both the client and the therapist (cf. Beneder 2011).

Classification runs the risk of meeting the client, 'from the outside,' as an expert who knows better and puts a label on the client's life problems in the form of a diagnosis. These labeling processes not only contribute to the stigmatization of mentally ill people in the community, but also to the fact that those labeled eventually follow the associated stereotypes and expectations in their behavior and even in their identity. The consequences of labelling can lead to more serious behavioral changes in the individual than the original disorder (for more details see Stemberger 2020).

Case Illustration

Finally, we will use a brief case description to illustrate the importance of GTP's assertion that *the clients must become their own diagnosticians* and how the therapist can support them in this process. For this purpose, we draw on the one hand on the therapist's notes and memories, and on the other hand on a final evaluation interview (tape recording, quotes are taken from the transcript) with the clients, in which they describe their experience of the initial phase of the therapy.

Situation of the client as recalled by the therapist

The client was in his mid-40s and lived an orderly life: successful in a secure job in a senior position, married for 15 years with two children. The reason for therapy was a gradually worsening difficulty in walking that increasingly confined him to bed. He was convinced that he was suffering from a neurological disease (amyotrophic lateral sclerosis, ALS), which leads to progressive paralysis of the muscles and is not curable according to current medical standards. All medical examinations resulted in negative findings, nevertheless his ability to walk became worse and worse. Due to this conviction, he could not believe the doctor's explanation that these phenomena had no physiological causes.

The therapist experienced the client as sympathetic, very focused on his physical experience, hardly noticing the other person, especially the therapist herself. He behaved in a friendly and open manner towards her, had hardly any expectations from her, not even of quick "successes" in the sense that his symptoms would improve as quickly as possible. Rather, he wanted a companion to help him deal with this serious illness. The therapist experienced the situation as one leaving a lot of room for maneuver, where one can look together sometimes in one direction and at other times in the other.

Situation of the client as he remembers it himself

He had exhausted himself professionally over the past 10 years, having been "Employee of the Year" several times. Professionally, he felt an imbalance between his effort and the reward he received from the company. But then came this walking disability. At first, he tried to ignore it, but there was no improvement. Since a distant relative had died of this disease (ALS), he gradually developed this self-diagnosis after he failed to improve his walking weakness despite rest and recuperation.

He was open to psychotherapy, as he had already had positive experiences with it, but not to a 'psychosomatic' explanatory model, which did not correspond at all to his self-image. He describes his first impression of the therapist as "the right mixture of caring, of catching me once, and a certain strength, in the sense of confidence, so that I had the impression: there is someone who is not immediately completely overwhelmed by my illness, which I experienced in real life, or who immediately puts it in the corner - everything is psychosomatic anyway, such a fantasy up there. It was important for me that I didn't have to be 'different' right away, that I didn't feel under pressure or that the therapist wanted to maneuver me in a direction that I didn't feel capable of going yet." The therapist's attitude of care, trust and confidence functioned as a guiding and holding force for the client from the beginning: "You had the necessary experience that there are very bad physical conditions that you can't make go away by snapping your fingers. And you conveyed to me that you are able to deal with it".

This example shows how important it is to recognize the client as his own diagnostician, even if one might be skeptical about his self-diagnosis. Rather, it was the therapist's task to deal respectfully with him and his self-diagnoses, and at first simply to 'do phenomenology' (cf. Böhm in this book). This open, respectful attitude of the therapist proved to be a supportive foundation for the client's further developmental steps, which enabled him to open up more and more and to explore himself. In this way, he gradually learned to establish a relationship with his body instead of viewing it only like an observer 'from the outside', as it were. Thus, step by step, he succeeded in perceiving and meeting his bodily needs by learning to care for himself more adequately. A further developmental step consisted in expanding his living space to the extent that he was also able to relate to the needs and demands of his social environment without immediately feeling overwhelmed. He learned to bring his own needs and requirements into a livable balance with those of others. In retrospect, he understood his life situation at that time as one of decision avoidance since the necessary professional changes only gradually became apparent. And as he puts it in his own words, "I didn't feel able to take any step – neither physical nor mental."

8. Gestalt Theoretical Psychotherapy – A Clinical Example

Thomas Fuchs[35]

Summary

The case of an anorectic patient is presented to demonstrate how well known symptomatic phenomena like a supposedly distorted body perception can be understood. Further theoretical suggestions are made to explain the motive to starve, without making complicated psychodynamic assumptions. To do so, genuine Gestalt theoretical concepts like „centering" and „reference system" are used. This leads to hints for a temporarily perception-focused formation of the therapeutic relationship.

Introduction

The aim of the paper is to outline some essentials of Gestalt Theoretical Psychotherapy (GTP) and how they contribute to a certain clinical approach. The case of a young woman with an eating disorder can illustrate the connection between a certain epistemological approach, theoretical assumptions concerning the perceptual level and clinical understanding of eating disorders and – emerging from these considerations – a certain conception of establishing the therapeutic bond.

Let us imagine a more or less typical[36] case of an anorectic young woman, 20 years old, student, and living in her own apartment since the beginning of her study one year ago, weighing 38kg with a body height of 168cm, which results in a body mass index of 13. So, this seems to be a severe case of anorexia – leaving aside for the moment other diagnostic criteria (Dilling & Freyberger 2016). The woman comes into therapy because there is pressure from her family and friends to do so, but her own initial commitment to therapy is low – rather typical for anorectic patients (Reich & Cierpka 2001, 73). They consider their starving often as a solution, not as a problem.

In dealing with anorexia nervosa, one has to answer these questions: what are the motives to starve? Why are starving, controlling nutrition and body-weight a solution for a psychic problem?

Often there are first answers on the biographical "surface": when she hit puberty, the young woman may have been a little bit overweight and someone made a remark: her sports coach, a teacher, a friend. Often one remark at a certain time, place, from a certain person can provoke the beginning of a

---

[35] Based on a lecture at the 21st Scientific Conference of the GTA "Motion – Spaces of Human Experience," 13th–15th June 2019, Warsaw, Poland, subsequently published in 2021 as an article in a special issue of the e-journal *Gestalt Theory*, 43(1), 87-99.

[36] Other phenomenal manifestations of anorectic disorders (e.g. in men, or in connection with sports in which body weight plays an important role) are not dealt with here.

starving process, at first typically accompanied by honouring comments. Then starving goes beyond a certain point and other people declare it no longer as "good-looking". However, the patient herself has already developed a need to starve. Starving "feels good", because it means being able to control something no one else can take over control.

What is suggested here is that the motive to starve is more or less the motive to gain control, because control got lost in the first place (which implies that control already played an important role because there is possibly no trust between the family members). In many cases, we're talking of loss of control over the role within the family (Bruch 2000), often characterised by a symbiotic relationship with the mother (Selvini Palazzoli 1984) and – due to marital problems of the parents and a forced compliance with the mother – an emotionally stressed relationship with the father (Buchholz & Dümpelmann 1993). Puberty plays an important part in this process, because it challenges the girl on different levels of cognitive and somatic developments: under these conditions leaving childhood and becoming a woman is threatening. So starving means in a way to stop this development – another possible motive (Boothe et al. 1993). By the beginning of the therapy, most patients are not aware of such motives to starve. All they know is that eating is threatening, it creates fear and panic.

These biographical details may have contributed to the anorectic development, but the current, present balance of field forces is always decisive for the maintenance of the symptomatology (Lewin 1936). In the here and now of the therapeutic encounter, the patient's outward appearance, including her gestures, facial expressions and manner of speaking, immediately comes to mind; it seems necessary for the therapist that the patient changes her eating habits as quickly as possible. This tempts anyone - as the above description of the symptoms shows - to reduce the patient to the anorectic symptomatology. This tendency is often supported by the patient herself - she seems to live in a world where everything is determined by diet and weight. Moreover, she lives - in the Central European cultural area - in a society where considerable moral pressure is exerted with regard to nutrition, fitness and appearance.

It is therefore a therapeutic challenge, especially at the beginning of treatment, to counteract this thematic narrowing. This is not done by ignoring what is obvious (and sometimes life-threatening), but by accepting, understanding and placing the symptoms in the patient's overall world. This can have a liberating effect, and if successful, the therapeutic encounter can become a model of how the patient can regain vitality precisely by (re)discovering sides of herself that are beyond a narrow world of control of food intake.

The following considerations will therefore concentrate on what seems to be the fruitful and distinguishing contribution of the Gestalt theoretical

116

approach to accept and understand the anorectic development in order to overcome the inherent narrowness.

The view on the patient´s body

In working with anorectic patients, every therapist is challenged by establishing a trustful therapeutic relationship. There is a pressure and ambivalence on both sides: The patient knows, that she can`t go on like this forever, but she feels the strong forces that will prevent her from eating enough. She simply cannot and will not give up control. This controlling side is experienced as an "inner critic" (cf. Henle 1962), who seems to be "harsh, unfair and without humanity" (p. 402). The therapist on the other side is confronted with the skinny body and the urgent demand that the patient has to gain weight for health reasons. Often the skinniness comes along with a deprived emotionality, a mimical depletion and a slowdown of movements which makes the whole expression of the patient kind of unlively: the patient obviously can´t care for herself, therefore a therapist is likely to adopt a helping and caring attitude and will be blind for the potentially encroaching effect on the patient. Or the patient will have an aggressive impact on the therapist in the first place, which often leads to more or less aggressive interventions like threatening the patient, forcing her to gain weight by therapy contracts or suggesting that the patient is not telling the truth.

But probably the most obvious conflict from the very beginning arises from the totally different perception of the patient`s body.

To begin with this last point:

We find the underlying phenomenon described in diagnostic manuals as "distorted body image" or "body scheme distortion" (Dilling & Freyberger 2016), which means that the patient will describe her skinny body as "fat", "too fat", "too big" etc.

The encounter between patient and therapist is therefore characterized by a different perception: In the phenomenal field of the therapist the patient has a skinny body. The patient herself states her body being too fat. This is illustrated in the following "egg-head"- picture:

What the patient states to be true

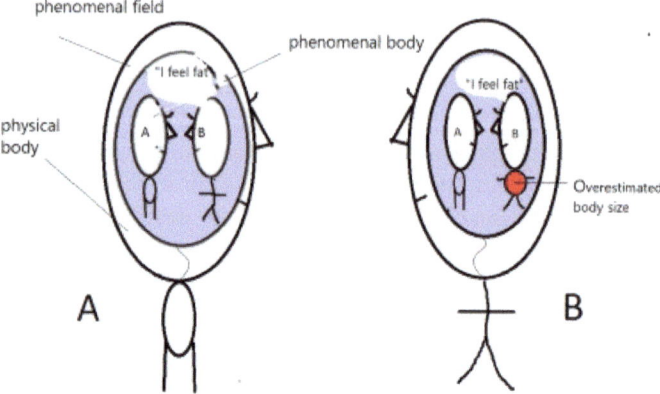

Fig. 1 The two „eggheads" representing the physical bodies of the therapist (A) and the patient (B) and their corresponding phenomenal fields coloured in violet. The statement of the patient („I feel fat") would indicate an overestimated body size (coloured in red). In the phenomenal field of the therapist both bodies appear in its more realistic dimensions.

One can ask now: does the patient really perceive (i.e. "see") her body as fat? Does she "feel" it? Or is she simply denying her own realistic perception by stating "fat" and actually seeing "thin"?

From what derives from a critical-realistic view (Sternek 2021), the perceived body is part of the phenomenal world. The own body is a perceived object like everything else. Perception can be distorted under certain conditions (very high or very low emotional arousal like being in love or suffering under pain or depressed feelings), but this will affect the whole phenomenal world: everything is coloured grey for the depressed person, the person with pain lives in a "painful" world (Stemberger & Sternek 2019). It is hardly possible that a single object of the perceived world is distorted while everything else appears to be of normal size and position. Therefore, it is very unlikely that an anorectic person perceives her own body as "fat", while all other persons are perceived in their normal size (Cash & Deagle 1997). If this is correct, then we can assume that anorectic patients are aware of the contradiction between her own perception and what they state about their body size. To put it short: they are aware that they are stating something that is not true. "Not true" is meant here in a critical-phenomenal sense (Bischof, 1966): the patient knows

118

intellectually, that it can`t be true. But she is experiencing something different (the so-called naïve-phenomenal view). Therefore it`s not a simple lie; patients can`t help themselves other than putting it this way (Fuchs 2010). When seeing for example a photography – especially with a friend beside her – the patient will "admit", that she is actually thin. All therapeutic interventions that lead to a reinforced body perception will therefore put the patient under stress, because she is confronted with this contradiction. Those interventions may be nevertheless helpful in therapy.

The following picture tries to show this:

What the patient knows to be true

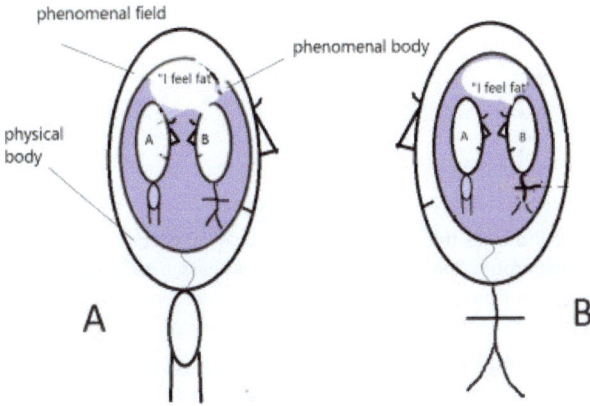

Fig. 2 The phenomenal fields of therapist and patient (coloured in violet) both indicate a realistic perception of the body sizes. The patient is aware of her skinniness in a critical-phenomenal sense, that means she knows she can`t be fat.

Patients suffer because of this contradiction and because of the everyday-pressure to live with it, because in almost all cases they themselves don`t understand why they have to state something that is definitely not true for the rest of the world. This contradiction has severe implications on an emotional level: a person who is experiencing something and who is aware of the fact that all others see and experience something totally different, will suffer from a very uncomfortable tension, often displayed by an inner restlessness.

But what the patients know to be true does not mean that their phenomenal worlds look like indicated in the picture shown before. There must be something else, which "forces" patients to state that they are feeling fat.

A possible theory explaining these phenomena can be derived from the following Gestalt theoretical assumptions: At some certain point or in a certain developmental phase in the life of the patient a "centering" (Galli 2010) occurred in the phenomenal field around the patient's perceived body. Many of us are familiar with cases of centering, for example, when we suffered an aching tooth. The tooth is small but the pain is big and so our whole phenomenal field will be cantered around this aching tooth.

First approach to what the patient is experiencing

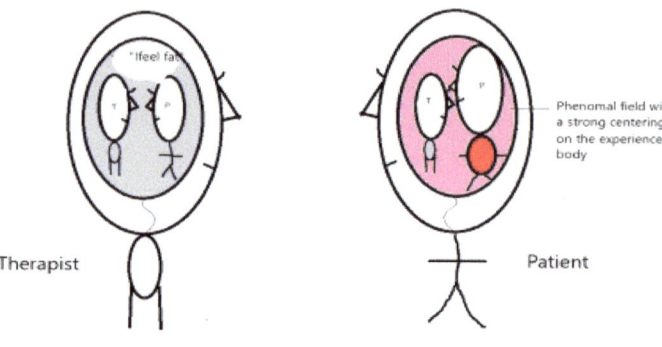

© Thomas Fuchs, ThomasFuchsPsycho@t-online.de

Fig. 3 The pink color indicates that the phenomenal field of the patient as a whole is affected by a centering around her body. She experiences herself as being „too present, too much, disturbing, not fitting" in the world she lives in and „translates" this experience as being „too fat" (overestimated body size coloured in red).

Presumably, the bodily changes in puberty together with the psychodynamic conflicts mentioned above may be responsible for this centering of the phenomenal field around the body. The young woman may experience the situation described above as being too present, too much, disturbing, not fitting anymore in the family constellation (or another social system). The accompanying feeling will be shame (Wurmser 1996). Shame as an emotion usually demands disappearing. However, at this time there will be no insight into such conflicts and no language to express them. As a consequence, the girl "translates" this experience as "being too fat" and the logically emerging method will be to start starving in order to turn back time, to undo the threatening bodily changes.

It is important to have in mind that motives to starve can change in the course of time. What has been a motive in the past, for example in puberty, must not be a motive in the presence. Often the experience that it "feels good" to control will lead to strong need to control with own demands even if the original social system with its strong impact for the girl has changed. It is likely

120

that the patient develops a compulsive manner with a high need to control and little trust in others that will influence new relationships in a way that intensity is avoided by keeping up a certain distance to others. It may be helpful for patient and therapist to have theories about possible motives in the past. For a successful process of change in therapy it is inevitable to look for the actual forces in the "here and now" in the phenomenal field of the patient.

Reference systems

The above mentioned "translation" of the experience of "being too present, not fitting" in "being too fat" needs further investigation. It can probably best be understood by analysing it in regard to the concept of reference system (dt.: Bezugssystem), which is central in the tradition of Gestalt theory (Metzger 2001; Galli & Trombini 2013). It deals with questions like: What refers to each other? What is the perspective on the reference system? What is constant, what is variable? Metz-Göckel investigated different variants of reference phenomena, including the so-called thematic field as a referring system. Different fields induce different meanings of an issue. (Metz-Göckel: „Die Bedeutung eines Sachverhalts ist durch das jeweilige Feld induziert", 2014, 364). A simple example for this could be words with a double meaning:

Prizes are too high in this exclusive shop!

Everybody`s won and all must have prizes!

The central referring system for the pubescent girl is her family. But if family dynamics look like suggested above (marital problems between the parents, a symbiotic relationship with the mother, a coerced betrayel of the father), important needs of the girl will not or not sufficiently be satisfied (needs for stability, safety, approval, the need to be understood etc.). Furthermore there are stress-enhancing duties: to be a partner for the mother, being responsible for a good atmosphere in the family, coping with the bodily and mental challenges in puberty.

In therapy it will be important to understand if a need, a wish, a goal has its origin in the patient or if it is induced by others (parents, peer-group, society). In any case: All this leads to an inner state of tension (Lindorfer 2021). In the experience of the girl this special and stressing role and the accompanying tension will be more or less self-evident, a given situation she grew up in. The potentially threatening forces emerging from this system will not be conscious. Therefore, these forces are functional – in opposite to phenomenal, experienced forces. Metz-Göckel: „Even if the fields can be made conscious, having thus phenomenal character, they often act only functionally, that means implicit or unconscious, having then in common with reference systems in the narrower sense their inconspicuousness. " (2014, 364; transl. ThF.)

The family system (or another social system) as a thematic field has a narrowing, demanding, paralysing effect. The „space of free movement" (Lewin 1940) is constricted, an effect of which the girl is not aware on a conscious level. Consciously perceptible and tangible are emotions like guilt, shame, fear and bodily sensations like exhaustion, strain, tiredness, narrowness. These emotions and sensations will coerce a switch. The family as the reference with the described demand character is fixed, is not changeable, so the girl inevitably is pushed to areas in which control and regulation are possible: Intellectual and sportive achievement (anorectic patients often are good pupils or students and sometimes sporty in a compulsive manner) and mainly dealing with one`s body and nutrition play a major part. Cultural impacts like the dominating ideal of beauty and morally charged notions about what is meant to be a healthy nutrition will strengthen these tendencies (Reich & v. Boetticher 2017).

The existentially important need of an ability to steer and control shifts from a (fixed, invariable) reference system of family relationships to a (better manageable, variable) reference system in topics like achievement, body, nutrition. The shift to another thematic field is experienced as a kind of liberation. This is why anorexia is seen as a solution, not as a problem.

Obviously, this liberation ends up in a new confinement: a phenomenal world dominated by (often compulsive) thoughts and behaviour concerned about weight and nutrition together with mental, bodily and social problems. That will lead to the segregation of a secondary total field (Tf_2) from the primary total field (Tf_1; cf. Stemberger 2009), a split which makes it possible to cope with all the tantalising effects of anorectic symptoms.

What the patient is experiencing

This centering of the body – like indicated in Fig. 3 and similar to Tf_1 in Fig. 4 - not only relates to the experienced body as an isolated part in the field, but the centering "colors" the entire field, it is a world dominated by one's own body. The unbearable experience of not fitting, disturbing, being too dominant is tied to the body. Starving should make the body disappear, or at least minimize its physical presence.

At the same time also applies - like sketched in Figure 2 - namely the patient's awareness of her actual (emaciated, painful, threatening) physical and (constricted, oppressive, overwhelming) mental state. This awareness is not lost, but it is incompatible with the control motive. This incompatibility is overcome by segregating a second phenomenal field.

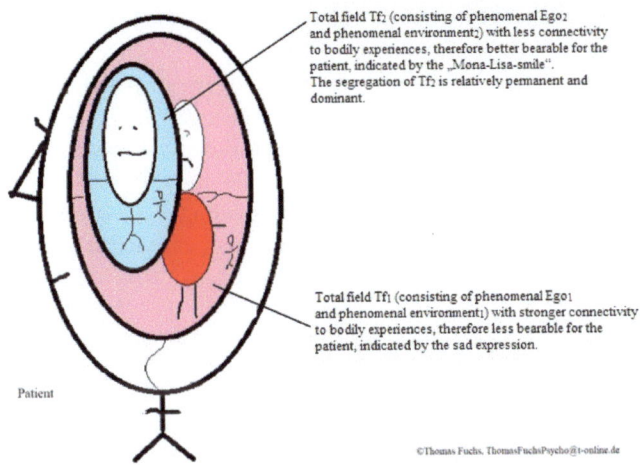

Total field Tf₂ (consisting of phenomenal Ego₂ and phenomenal environment₂) with less connectivity to bodily experiences, therefore better bearable for the patient, indicated by the „Mona-Lisa-smile". The segregation of Tf₂ is relatively permanent and dominant.

Total field Tf₁ (consisting of phenomenal Ego₁ and phenomenal environment₁) with stronger connectivity to bodily experiences, therefore less bearable for the patient, indicated by the sad expression.

Patient

©Thomas Fuchs, ThomasFuchsPsycho@t-online.de

Fig. 4 Segregation of a second phenomenal total field Tf₂

Such segregation always takes place when circumstances arise that are incompatible as a whole[37]. This usually happens completely informally and automatically, e.g. when reading a book, during a film showing in the cinema, when visiting the theater: the primary phenomenal field with more physiological anchoring ("I sit in the cinema seat and look at a screen") moves into the background, a second phenomenal field of a more virtual nature (I become an active participant in a captivating film plot) dominates my experience. When the lights turn on again in the cinema, the secondary total field collapses and I am back in an undivided primary total field. The lawfulness of such processes was described by Rausch (1982) in connection with looking at images and transferred to psychotherapeutic processes by Stemberger (2009).

Elsewhere (Fuchs 2010, 2014) the assumption was made that anorectic patients develop a second phenomenal field relatively permanently, because this is the only way to endure the painful and threatening physical and mental states. This also explains why the confrontation with their own body (physical exercises, mirrors, photos, films) are very uncomfortable for the patients because they are then forced to switch to their first phenomenal field.

Not the phenomenon as such, but the persistence of the segregation and the relative dominance of Tf₂ over Tf₁ is to be recognized as a significant pathological characteristic of anorexia. Mere weight gain will do little to change that. We must therefore agree with Bruch, who recognized as early as 1962:

---

[37] A general introduction to the Multiple-Field-Approach is given in Stemberger 2022b.

"Without a corrective change in the body image, however, the improvement is apt to be only a temporary remission."

Such a correction means that the patient can endure her own body in terms of the first phenomenal total field.

However, this will only be the case when it - as described above - can no longer be experienced as "disruptive" or "not suitable" in the overall frame of reference. This, however, requires a deeper understanding of the effective systemic forces and the entire underlying psychodynamics in order to better understand and experience one's own position in the system.

Hints for a therapeutic strategy

In working with anorectic patients, some of Metzger's "characteristics of working at the living" (Metzger 1962/2022, Böhm 2021) become a demanding and challenging sound, for example: "Shaping the process by using the forces inherent within the living being" (Metzger 1962/2022, transl. Böhm 2021, also in this volume) Böhm states: "psychotherapy will only succeed when it is based on the forces acting within the patient." This may appear kind of absurd in dealing with anorectic patients, but there is a deeper truth in it nonetheless. For therapy with anorectics, this is a first initial strategy: Supporting the patient by helping her to understand what she is doing and that there is a certain logic in what she is doing. The implied messages may be: "You are not crazy and you're not a liar and I accept that you have to state that you 'feel' fat."

In working with anorectic patients, it can be useful to highlight this contradiction right from the beginning of the therapy process. It can be done – more or less – by explaining to the patient what has been explained here. It's not that difficult to understand and in almost all cases, anorectic patients are quite smart and intelligent – so that will help too.

That implies a kind of perception-cantered strategy at the beginning of therapy, but it will possibly help the patient to approach the strong affective side of her problem. The explanations concerning critical realism and perception will help the patient to understand her inner conflict on a perceptual level and why it implies that she feels ashamed.

It is definitely useless to argue with the patient intellectually about what is right and what is wrong, neither on the topic of nutrition or gaining weight nor on the topic of body perception. The aim suggested here is to establish an atmosphere in which "it is allowed" to speak out loudly what she is experiencing. At this point the therapist has a very important task that has to come along with his empathic efforts: Supporting the patient to find the right words that can express what she is experiencing. If it's true that most of effectual forces are functional, that means not conscious, we can't expect that there is an established language that helps to discover, to name and to express the sensations and emotions accompanying the exploration of her phenomenal world. That means for therapists to take over a rather active position. The next step has to be to find out more about the possible motives to starve. However, this will hopefully happen under the condition that the patient feels more accepted and more understood and is motivated to further explore her phenomenal world. In common with a certain therapeutic attitude (Böhm 2021) this perception-cantered strategy can facilitate empathic processes: not only for the therapist in understanding the world of the patient, but also vice versa. By feeling understood the patient may gradually adopt the therapist's way to "look" at the patient's inner world (cf. Fuchs 2020). This requires an empathic effort by the patient which will possibly alter the perspective on herself and others and modify the harsh attitude of her inner critic (Henle 1962, 402).

9. Reconciliation of Time Perspectives as a Criterion for Therapy Completion

Giancarlo Trombini in collaboration with Elena Trombini and Gerhard Stemberger[38]

Summary

Giancarlo Trombini presents the continuation of his research on the question of which criteria can be used to assess the progress of therapy in an objectively verifiable way and to make the decision on the completion of therapy. In the first phase of his research, the phenomenological criterion of a qualitative change in the patient's relations towards the positive and towards higher complexity was proposed for this purpose. In terms of the working method in analytic therapy, this meant concretely: attention should be paid to what development is shown in the comparison of the relationships that occur in the dream narrative and in the subsequent associations. This criterion was therefore given the name MDAC - comparison between the manifest dream and the subsequent associations. The idea can easily be transferred to those therapy methods which do not primarily work with reports of dream memories and subsequent associations - also in other ways of working it is possible to pay attention in the way suggested by Trombini to the qualitative development of the relationships which are thematized by the clients in the course of an hour.

To this first criterion, another phenomenological criterion is now added in the present paper: that of the "concluding therapeutic turn" (CTT). If the patient's development reaches this turn in the course of the therapy in one session, this indicates, according to Trombini, that the therapy can soon be concluded. The fulfillment of this criterion can be recognized by the fact that in the sequence of dream narration and subsequent associations in a session a relational dynamic towards the positive and towards higher complexity becomes recognizable and that is at the same time connected with a reconciliation of the three temporal reference systems (past, present, future). The achievement of this "concluding therapeutic turn" indicates that the patient is aware of the changes made in

[38] This work is dedicated to the memory of our friends Anna Arfelli Galli and Giuseppe Galli. The principal author is especially grateful to them for encouraging him to supplement his medical training with one as a Gestalt psychologist and psychoanalyst. The major part of the text was originally written in Italian by the main author, Giancarlo Trombini, in cooperation with Elena Trombini. Some supplementary references to German-language literature and corresponding concepts of Gestalt theory and Gestalt Theoretical Psychotherapy (GTP) in the first chapters were added by Gerhard Stemberger at the invitation of the main author. Elena Trombini and Gerhard Stemberger provided for the present English-language version. This English version was first published in 2021 in a special issue of the e-journal *Gestalt Theory*, 43(1), 101-119; a German version appeared a year before, 2020, in the journal *Phänomenal*, 12(2), 33-44, under the title "Vergangenheit, Gegenwart und Zukunft als Bezugssystem. Die Versöhnung der Zeitperspektiven als Kriterium für den Therapieabschluss".

therapy, and at the same time makes it clear to the therapist that the therapy is nearing completion.

Introduction

Giancarlo Trombini, the main author of this paper, has demonstrated in a series of empirical studies based on treatment examples from psychoanalytic psychotherapy that the development of relational dynamics in therapy can be assessed in an objectively verifiable way using a phenomenological criterion based on the narrative content of each session. This criterion is the comparison between the manifest dream and the subsequent associations (MDAC[39]; Trombini 2010; 2014; 2015). This is a contribution to the reflexive pole of analytic psychotherapy, which is, after all, characterized by a constant oscillation between the pole of reflection and the pole of a "dreaming reception". The present contribution continues this research with the treatment of the concluding phase of therapy, which is related to certain turning points in the processes of change in therapy (Di Chiara 2003). As a complement to the MDAC criterion, another phenomenological criterion is now presented here: that of the "concluding therapeutic turn" (CTT)[40]. This indicates that the patient[41] is about to complete the therapy. At this turn, as will be explained in the following, in a successful case the reconciliation of the three temporal frames of reference (the psychological past, the psychological present, the psychological future) can be observed in a single session. This shows that the patient is sufficiently aware of the changes that have taken place in her to be able to conclude the therapy soon - also in the knowledge of the associated separation from the therapist.

In the previous works it was suggested to objectively check the progress of therapy on the basis of MDAC criterion: The qualitative development of the relationships occurring in the dream narratives and the subsequent associations to the positive or negative, to higher or lower complexity makes the development of the relationship dynamics visible in a factually verifiable way. Following a suggestion by Stemberger[42], the development of the patient's

---

[39] The abbreviation MDAC stands for "manifest dream/association comparison", in Italian the abbreviation is CSMA.

[40] In Italian, the "snodo terapeutico conclusivo", STC.

[41] Since all the patients mentioned in this article are women and the analyst is a man, the corresponding gender designations are used. In the relevant statement, all genders are meant in each case.

[42] This suggestion was based on considerations by Mary Henle (1962), which are translated into a threefold relationship centering in Gestalt Theoretical Psychotherapy GTP (Stemberger 2018a): GTP focuses in a pendulum movement once on the interpersonal relationships of the patient in everyday life, then again on the therapeutic relationship with the therapist, but then also on the relationship of the patient to herself. It is

inner-personal relationship, i.e. her relationship to herself, should now also be included with the help of the CTT criterion. We want to consider this inner-personal relationship of the patient on the basis of her psychological time perspective, i.e., her past, her present, and her future; past, present, and future not in the historical but in the psychological sense (cf. Lewin 1951[43]). In the relation to her past, present and future, the relation of a person to herself is shown quite essentially. The CTT criterion must be seen together with the MDAC criterion, since the development of the relationship dynamic to other persons cannot be separated from the development of the relationship dynamic of the person to herself, as expressed in the frame of reference of the time perspective in the patient's life space. We assume that a development towards more positive and complex interpersonal relationships of the patient must go hand in hand with her "reconciliation" with her past, present and future. In the successful case, this dynamic develops positively as a whole in the course of the therapeutic sessions.

Contemporary psychoanalysis assumes that the relational structures in the dream narrative reveal the structures of the person's "inner world" (Ogden 2009; Blum 2011). For psychoanalysis, changes in the manifest content of the dream are clear indications of transformations of object relations in the unconscious world (Leuzinger-Bohleber, 2018). Dream and associations are parts of a whole, the analytic session must be interpreted as a whole, in a sense like one big dream (Carloni 1991).

The therapist explores together with the suffering patient her pain with the aim that through it she regains the ability to overcome negative (destructive) relationships and to cultivate new positive (constructive) relationships that are accessible to her. In the successful case, she should be enabled again to realize in her relationships those forms of with-human interaction that Giuseppe Galli calls "social virtues" (Galli 2005). For this purpose, the analyst offers the patient the possibility to unfold her transference process without encountering a countertransference that hinders her, instead of supporting her in her search for the truth (Di Chiara 2003).[44]

---

assumed that there are dynamic interactions between these three relationship spheres that can be addressed therapeutically.

[43] "The totality of the individual's views of his psychological future and his psychological past existing at a given time may be called 'time perspective' (L.K. Frank 1939)." (Lewin 1951, 75). For further research on the psychological implications of time perspective, see Nuttin & Lens 1985 and Stolarski, Fieulaine & van Beek 2015.

[44] For the specific understanding of transference and countertransference in Gestalt Theoretical Psychotherapy, see Kästl 2007.

To assess the transformative relational dynamics reflected in the content of a session's narratives (which, of course, cannot be separated from the relational dynamics between patient and therapist), the MDAC criterion considers two categories:

The basic category is that of *positivity/negativity of the relationships* the narratives are about and their development from the dream narrative to the subsequent associations. This category is considered an indicator of either progressive, regressive, or stagnant development in therapy. One compares the relational structures of the characters that appear in the manifest (phenomenal) content of the dream narrative in the particular session (as an expression of an intrapsychic experience that becomes an interpersonal one) with the relational structures of the characters that appear in the subsequent associations. These associations shed light on the emotional-dreamlike atmosphere of the moment (Bezoari & Ferro 1992). Comparing the dream narrative with the subsequent associations, one thus follows the developmental trajectory of the relational dynamics that emerge in the particular session.

The second category of the MDAC criterion is that of *relational complexity*; this is inextricably linked to the category of positivity. In fact, a relationship dynamic that develops in the direction of increased complexity (such as the transition from a dyadic to a triadic relationship) can only be considered positive if the session itself comes to a positive conclusion. The idea of relational dynamics moving toward increased complexity is inherent in the developmental notion of the therapeutic model of psychoanalysis (Falci 2005; De Toffoli 2008; Trombini 2014) as well as in the Prägnanz principle of Gestalt psychology (Rausch 1966) and Gestalt Theoretical Psychotherapy that builds on that principle. A clear and concise account of the category of relational dynamics in psychotherapy was recently presented by Stemberger (2018).

The MDAC criterion can be used to identify the progressive or regressive tendency of a session's relationship dynamics or its tendency to stagnate. The results of the different sessions can also be compared in this respect. Thus, it is possible to assess what happens in the different stages (initial, intermediate, final) of the therapy. Clinical examples have already been used to highlight the concrete signs of change in the relationship dynamics between the beginning of therapy and the completion stage (Trombini 2014, 2015). This change, as has been shown, is accompanied by symptomatic improvement and by the observable acquisition of analytic competencies by the patient (in the sense of Bolognini 2008). Thus, the MDAC criterion is essentially an instrument for the assessment of progress in the development of the psychotherapeutic field (for a review, see Trombini, Corazza & Stemberger 2019).

Thus, paying attention to changes in the relational constellations in the manifest narratives in therapy deepens the awareness of the progress of the therapeutic process, which in the analyst is fed by the sources of evenly-suspended attention, empathy, countertransference, and the widest possible grasp of all connections.

Research hypotheses

The research that initially led to the development of the MDAC criterion is now continuing.

The therapeutic process, starting from the present of the therapeutic relationship, grasps the whole time perspective, breaks free from the fruitless repetitions, opens to the future and can accept the past (Balsamo 2019). The time perspective places every relational event in therapy in a temporal frame of reference (past, present, future). When the patient has reconciled with her psychological present and her psychological past, and thus transformed them as well, a hopeful view of the future is also possible.

Such a happening, as we can observe in the concluding phases of therapies, is manifested in what we call the "concluding therapeutic turn" (CTT) of the transformation process. At this turning point, the patient is already aware of the path she has taken to such an extent that she can think of concluding the therapy. Retrospection and transformation now distinguish who she was then from who she is now (Di Chiara 2003). The patient prepares herself for separation, for the conclusion of the analysis, able to let go and ready to be let go (Bigi 2004).

According to Metzger (2001, 140), the person with all her relationships can only be understood in each case from her relationship to a frame of reference, "as the area in which he or she is located and moves, in which he or she has his or her place, direction, and measure" (cf. on this Metz-Göckel 2014; Sternek 2020). The frame of reference can express itself in different settings and can itself undergo changes, which in turn bring about changes in the experience and behavior of the person concerned. In this context, Metzger also refers to the importance of embedding life in the passage of time. Accordingly, in the present work we turn to the temporal frames of reference of the past, present, and future.

Some time ago we already presented a clinical case in which the time perspective was interpreted as a frame of reference in psychotherapy (Galli & Trombini 2013). From the continuation of the related considerations grew the idea that this could be a possible criterion for whether the patient has already become sufficiently aware of the path of change she has embarked upon. Once this awareness is developed, it can result in a session that already carries the therapy conclusion within itself, even if it is not yet explicitly agreed upon at that time. This is then a session of the "concluding therapeutic turn." Such a session is characterized by the accomplishment of a reconciliation of the temporal frames of reference (psychological past, present, future) in the contents of the dream narrative and the subsequent associations, while at the same time maintaining favorable relational dynamics in the sense of the MDAC criterion.

In a concise way, this criterion of the "concluding therapeutic turn" is fulfilled when a progessive relational dynamic is embedded in the patient's temporal frames of reference in such a way that there is a transition from understanding the past (represented in the dream narrative as a conflictual underlying problem) to a positive experience of the present that has made peace with the past and is open to a hopeful view of the future.

Starting with the "sample case" for this research hypothesis, already published in Galli & Trombini 2013 and in Galli 2017, four clinical case studies will now be presented to allow an assessment of the fertility of the new proposal.

Four clinical cases

First case

At the age of 40 the patient asked for psychological help as she was troubled by the exacerbation of a psychosomatic disorder (a rosaceous erythema) localized to the face, which sometimes would cause her an unbearable burning sensation. She also felt desperate: a state that had progressively worsened one year after the death of her mother. At the beginning of the analysis she revealed her desperate sense of isolation with a dream: "I am locked up motionless in a coffin underground". In the dream her depressive condition is expressed by the coffin that suffocates her vitality.

She felt a sense of inner emptiness, as disclosed by a dream in which a blue strand came out of her open body, devoid of internal organs, which for the therapist was a clear reference to the "Telefono Azzurro" (Blue Phone children's helpline), an Italian association which acts to tackle the problem of maltreatment and abuse to children. She could no longer bear her husband, whom for a long time she had found selfish and insensitive, unlike the first period of their relationship, but whom she did not leave for the love of her daughter.

She had established an idealized relationship with her mother, since the age of three and a half. In fact, her father had been admitted to a psychiatric hospital, where he remained for the rest of his life as, following a psychotic crisis, he threatened to stab his wife, his daughter and his one-year-old son. A tragic event that will be painfully printed on her face with the erythema. A face that requires gentle caresses. From six to fourteen years, her mother had entrusted her to a college run by nuns for the school periods and to family relatives for most of the holidays.

Now we will see a session of the last phase of the psychotherapy.

The patient tells a dream: "I am in a convent of nuns. At the windows there are metal grills. In that convent there are the novices that will then go missionaries. A nun approaches and gives me a blank booklet ". The patient says that the booklet given by the nun is like the one she received for her first communion and confirmation. It is the pleasant memory of an initiation ceremony in which the bishop gives her the chrism: Occurrence in which she received the booklet. She says than that the convent with the metal grills reminds her of a prison and of a psychiatric hospital. For her father the psychiatric hospital became a prison for life.

The therapist has here the opportunity to tell her that her relationship with him in his maternal function, represented by the nun, is integrated with that of his paternal function, always expressed by him and represented by the bishop, so that she can go out into the world and not remain imprisoned in the therapy transformed into a convent-prison-psychiatric hospital. The session ends with her saying:

"It's a pity the booklet they gave me is blank, nothing is written on it". The patient is here attempting a depressive reaction.

The therapist says: "Everything has yet to be written"

The patient: "I had not thought about it (an expression that is the "yes" of the unconscious). This is beautiful".

With the expression "this is beautiful" she shows her disposition to overcome her actual problem, which is represented by the conflict between remaining protected in the convent-psychotherapy or leaving this situation, attracted by a condition of autonomy and by recognizing her capacity to implement the separation and reach a position of separateness. The patient's sufficient awareness of the transformative path taken is a prelude to her imminent and adequate request to conclude the therapy, with which she had overcome the problem of facial burning, the sense of despair and developed a sense of meaningfulness of her own experience (her "mission").

We can now consider the last phase of the psychotherapy on the light of the temporal frames of reference, bearing in mind its location, its changes and the relationships that arise from it.

The booklet, which the therapist-nun gives to the patient, can contain everything that has been thought and written by the couple patient-therapist during the many therapeutic sessions. This booklet represents the result of the work done in the past until today. It is the history of the therapy seen in the frame of reference of the past.

Then the frame of reference changes. The patient has become a novice who will go into the world (a world that offers her a reconciled relationship with her

132

husband and in which she can find comfort through the love for her daughter). The booklet is presented in the frame of reference of the presence as a passport to leave the convent, so that it does not turn into a prison-mental hospital. In the frame of reference of the past the patient participated in an initiation rite together with the therapist-bishop, as witnessed by the booklet. It is for her the confirmation of the possible transition to autonomy. In the frame of reference of the present she has a booklet with which she can get started in life. She will have to enter a "new world" and now consults her booklet as a possible guide. Unfortunately, she finds out that nothing is written there. It is blank and this depresses her. Here the therapist offers a different frame of reference pointed toward the future. In this frame of reference, the booklet has yet to be written. The patient accepts with pleasure the frame of reference proposed by the therapist. She has gained confidence in herself and in others and feels hopeful for the life that awaits her.

Therefore, in one single session the patient undergoes various temporal transitions with connected transformations of her emotional state. She overcomes the feeling of despair of the frame of reference of the past and in the frame of reference of the present the booklet appears as a symbol of openness to her actual life. In the frame of reference of the future the booklet transforms into a symbol of hope and trust shared with her therapist. The booklet can be read as the "other self" with whom the patient finds herself in a dynamic relationship that evokes the history of the therapeutic couple. At the same time, the booklet announces the internal dialogue that, in her life "in mission", she will continue with the introjected figure of her therapist. In conclusion, the interpretation of the temporal perspective as frame of reference during the psychoanalytic treatment allows us to highlight that the ability to make a transition from the understanding of the past to the open present to a hopeful future in the same session is the concluding turn of the analysis. What we observed so far on the simultaneous transit of the three temporal frames of reference is in agreement with their dynamic relationship. At first, in her dream, we see a dyadic relationship structure (the patient and the nun) that is, though, of an undefined quality. This relationship acquires a positive quality in the associations where the positive relationship with the bishop also appears. A triadic relationship (positive and complex) is, therefore, organized: The patient with the nun and the bishop who gave her the booklet. Finally, the associations end with a positive monadic position of openness to a trustful future. The therapeutic process is close to completion.

Second case

The patient, in her twenties, asked for a psychoanalytic treatment because she suffered from compulsive bulimic attacks. She criticized her mother for over-feeding all family members: her, her younger brother (the parent's favorite) and even her husband. The father, obese, carried out his flourishing working activity with intelligence and business sense while lying in bed. During the analysis the patient normalizes her eating behavior by reaching and maintaining an adequate weight. However, she laments a sense of emptiness, a depressing difficulty in facing sacrifices, and the inability to make the decision to live alone. During the therapy, reflecting on her ambivalent desire for separation, she questions her filial attitudes and her inexhaustible demands. Over time she manages to gradually separate from her family. At first, she carves out a personal area in her father's house where she can live. Later she moves in her own apartment, but her mother keeps on supplying and filling her with food. She complains of psychosomatic pains in various part of her body, especially in her legs, for which she refers to a physiotherapist. It gives her anxiety to walk on her feet on her own path. For this reason, she spends a lot of time at home, in bed. Finally, she builds a relationship with a stable partner. The psychosomatic pains reduce until they disappear.

We present now some aspects of the final period of the analysis. She informs the analyst that she carried out several tasks during the week: She accompanied her father to a medical checkup, on her own initiative; she helped the maid with housework; she offered herself to occasionally look after her brother's son, a willingness never before granted.

Next, this session appears.

Patient: "What a change after all these years! For the first time I organized a birthday party for my partner inviting people at home. I cooked by myself without using mum's cooked food. So far, I had always warmed her food up. I have seen mum doing things and now I have become quite capable. In the past I valued just the appearance of things, now I am more interested in the substance, the internal aspect. How much importance I once gave to an extra kilo of weight!"

She tells a dream: I went to the church of S. Luca, what a nice place! (the church of S. Luca is on the hill above Bologna. In this church there is the effigy of the Virgin, much venerated in the city and destination for pilgrims). Now, passing various obstacles I have to enter the city. I take several busses. I pass through beautiful roads that I do not know. I start walking again like it is in reality. What a joy to be able to walk: It means standing alone. San Luca: I was helped by the Virgin!

She comments: "the Virgin is a mother. Psychoanalysis is too. I got stuck in my life and I could not walk. I was so dependent on my mother! I did not want to lose her. Now I am quite successful in doing by myself.

Therapist: "it is a good starter dream"

Patient: "I hope so, but there is also the fear of not making it alone. But I think I will keep with me the bond with you, who have changed me with affection".

In the manifest material of both the dream and the associations the patient has achieved a personal positive state. She has learned to making it alone and to manage living with her partner. She is close to the end of the treatment. She is confident that she will be able to treasure inside an affectionate couple relationship with her therapist, to maintain a position of potential closeness in the future separation.

We can see that the patient can now summarize with understanding how she was in the temporal frame of reference of the past and how old events affect the present. The frame of reference of the present shows us how the patient is now: She has improved her sense of self-esteem. Thus, she opens up to the frame of reference of the future in the confident hope of knowing how to manage it personally and with autonomy.

We know that the concluding phase of the analysis can disclose itself with dreams of crossing borders, of concluding travels, of acquiring spaces, and, as in the preset case, of entering the city (Masciangelo, 1987; Di Chiara, 2003). The session became a concluding therapeutic turn.

Third case

The patient, as she was close to forty years, asked for an analysis as she was suffering from several somatization problems (headache, irritable bowel syndrome, fibromyalgia, palpitation). She had a hypochondriac attitude, sometimes culminating in intense death anxieties that began shortly after marriage. These symptoms seriously worsen after the loss of her mother, a person of very poor health, reason why in her family she had always felt an anguished expectation of death.

She felt like an unwanted daughter as the mother got pregnant believing she was sterile. The mother, without any passion agreed to marry the cousin of the man she loved in vain. The patient had no memories of loving moments with her mother. Since it was necessary to save money, given the uncertain health of her mother, she was often forced to play only with her father's work tools (which was done at home) that were given to her instead of the desired toys. She disdained her father and called him stingy in attitudes and feelings. Her husband, in her opinion, had always been faithful to her. However, unlike what happened in the premarital period, she rarely indulged with her husband during the marriage and when she did it was usually without pleasure. She complained that her husband was "really present" and "caring" only when she was ill (as was often the case) and accompanied her to medical examinations. Instead, she described as optimal the relationship with her daughter.

In the first phase of the analysis, she spends most of time describing her symptoms, as typical of psychosomatic patients, considered to be signs of scaring deadly illnesses. Lately she develops curiosity for symbolic aspects as she can feel that her body is seen and imagined by her analyst. Signs of psychological developments appears. The patient starts to integrate in a useful way the experiences of exclusion and jealousy. This is associated with the clear psychic ability to express herself in a more vivid way and in knowing how to nurture the hope of future pleasant moments. The psychosomatic symptoms and the death anxiety disappear. The patient finds the internal strength to resume her work. Unfortunately, this development is interrupted: she misses an opportunity for an important job. It is a bitter failure that tremendously upsets her and provokes significant changes in her behavior. She gets rid of her usual social relationships and isolate herself as much as possible from her husband and her daughter. This behavior leads to her husband's angry outburst and to the gradual estrangement of her daughter. Later she develops new relationships that lead her to suddenly take distance from her family and from the analysis. She promises to return but she then does not.

This behavior elicits my disappointment, anger, and the phantasy that she will interrupt the analysis. The analyst's capacity to survive and communicate is severely put to the test. Reflected in the transference and countertransference, the feeling of not existing for the other (experienced by the patient in her life and by the analyst now) takes on clear evidence. This helps the analyst to rediscover the necessary affection toward this person so devastated by the contingences of her life. Gradually, the compulsion to stay away from the meetings dissipates. Meanwhile, her daughter prematurely found work in a distant location. The anxiety of losing her strengthen. The sweet memories of them having breakfast at the bar returns. She plans to contact her daughter and she is warmly supported by her husband in this, with whom she has now rediscovered the intimacy they had during the premarital period.

On the occasion of her daughter's return home, she tides her toys up in her room and decorates the windows with colorful butterflies, but she then fears the daughter might not appreciate it. Thus, she opens the following session.

Dream: "I was in my daughter's room, but the window was no longer colored. Black shadows were visible. So sad! I get closer: They are swallows". Then, she complains: "What a bad dream I had! I am lonely and sad".

This is the feeling of loneliness that characterized her life from childhood onwards. The joy of seeing her daughter again and being together pleasantly (golden butterflies) disappears at the thought of the emptiness she will see in her room after her departure. The analyst thinks the patient wonders when she will see her daughter again: perhaps it will be a long undefined sad wait.

Suddenly the analyst recalls a good memory of when the patient was talking about her summers at the beach with her baby daughter. Punctually, with pleasure, she saw the swallows reappear every year. It also happened that one day one of them made a nest under their veranda. It seems appropriate to the analyst to intervene.

Analyst: "the swallows return in spring".

Patient: "spring... the return... I had not thought about it. This is beautiful. Even children are swallows when they feel the desire to be together with their parents".

Analyst: "it is a flowering that reappears every year".

Patient: "it can be counted on to happen... My daughter is back, she was satisfied with the way I had arranged her room... She thanked me with a smile".

On that occasion the patient was able to pleasantly chat, together with her husband, with her daughter about her future work and love projects: She savored feeling part of the familiar We. The analyst feels they are approaching to the concluding part of the treatment.

In the dream and in the subsequent associations the patient is in a monadic negative state. However, later, through the associative exchange between the analyst and the patient, the relational dynamic develops positively. In the psychoanalytic field a satisfying dyadic relationship comes into shape and transforms into a pleasant triadic relationship. Therefore, in the material of the session a progressive relational dynamic, according to the categories of positivity and degree of complexity, is perceived. The transformations of the meaning of the swallows in the dream are also grasped in the light of the temporal collocation. When they are black shadow, in the frame of reference of the past, they can be a symbol of the depression that characterized the patient's history. When they are shadow shallows, in the frame of reference of the present, they become a symbol of the return of her daughter. Finally, the swallows evoke the spring that will always return. It is the frame of reference toward the future in confident expectation. The patient is now aware of her acquired capacity to be left and let go her daughter and her husband when necessary. The concluding therapeutic turn took place. The patient experiences this transit that occurs in the temporal perspective passing from the memory of the past to the perception of the present and then to the hope in the future as a coherent unit, a harmonious whole. In fact, she will soon finish the therapy with satisfaction.

Fourth case

The patient, twenty years old, a graduate nurse, asked for an analysis because she could not find the courage to begin a hospital attendance. She defined herself as introvert and fearful in social relationships. For a long time, this was also the case in the therapeutic relationship. The description of her life and the expression of her feelings required a lot of clinical patience from the therapist.

With her brother, two years younger than her, she was raised with love by the paternal grandmother, who was rather apprehensive about their health. Meanwhile, their parents completed their university studies in another city. The patient, in the initial school life, describes herself as a child who was "petrified" while she saw the other children move with ease. By the end of the high school, she had talked only to half of the class. She describes the relationship with her mother as symbiotic so that "everything that was outside of that small area with mum was terrifying". After high school, with "difficulty", she enrolled in the nursing school of her town: "the spirit of the Red Cross nurse prevailed in me".

The mother thought she should go the University and then move away from her hometown like her parents had done. She became so got angry at her husband for not guiding their daughter in the best possible way. The mother had been inhibited by her father from gaining experience abroad and she often complained about this to her daughter. The patient said: "I have her experiences within me as if they were mine because she repeated them to me countless times".

After a long initial period of analysis, the patient was finally able to undertake her nursing activity at the hospice for elderly women (the grandmothers). Later, she managed to move away from the hospice and decided to attend the hospital emergency room, where she was later hired. There she met an elderly colleague (a paternal substitute) who helped her a lot and with whom she lived for several years.

Gradually, during her analysis she understood her "unexploded anger" toward her parents and the mental confusion that often dominated her and that she expressed through obsessive-phobic symptoms. She became an appreciated nurse, and her psychic symptoms began to lessen. She progressively implemented various separations. At first, she left her partner, who would have liked to continue living with her. She then took a sufficient distance from her parents, who were constantly asking for her presence. She understood that moving away from them did not mean abandoning them: A daughter is not obliged to give back to her parents all the time they have dedicated to her.

The father began, more and more often, to ask her for health advice for her mother, who was really sick, but then he did not accept her suggestions. He rejected the advice saying: "mom is not that bad". This defense of the father, that is, not wanting to admit that his wife's health was deteriorating, was not perceived by the daughter, who, on the contrary felt not appreciated in her medical competence.

138

The progress of the analysis allowed the growth of a creative aspect of her: Writing fairy tales accompanied by images with watercolors that she herself created. This creativity signaled the beginning of the conclusion of the analysis. In this final stage the patient opens the session with a dream:

"I am with you (the therapist) at the bar, sitting at a small table. I speak to you, who are a notary. I list you that we have already seen this, that and the other. At one point I tell you that we have talked enough. I get up and walk away. I approach a hairdresser, who is there at the bar and start asking him questions". She comments: "It is strange that I ask questions to the hairdresser. It's a sad dream, but in the dream I was not sad".

The analyst thinks that the notary-therapist certifies the list of separations that have taken place and those to be completed. The meeting with the hairdresser, who styles and embellishes what is on the surface of the head, documents the acquired ability to handle what is visible, the conscious emerged from the depth. This is what the analyst tells her.

The patient agrees and then goes on to talk about her great need for sweets, and the excessive number of people at the bar. She complains of her father: "He seems to ask but then he wants to decide by himself what to do for mum. I eat too much even though I am not hungry because of the frustration of my father that gets on my nerves". So, at this point she accepts the therapist's comment about her father: "he does not want to see his wife's physical decay worsen". She also adds: "Dad gives now grate proof of his love for mum". Finally, she concludes the session by informing the therapist that she has started a new tale about the sea: It talks about the relationship between a child and his mother.

Patient: "it is astonishing how much writing captivates me! Perhaps it is a continuation of the analysis. I am really fond of these little creatures (the characters from the fairy tales)"

Therapist: "these are the characters you have inside"

Patient: "yes, they have something magical. However, why do I eat so much?"

Therapist: "You wait to be fed by the characters of the fantasy. Everyone must find his own way to continue the analysis".

It might be enlightening to report some concluding passages from the fairy tale that the patient told the therapist a year earlier. A fairy tale the patient is now trying to get published by a publishing house.

This child, Isaac, an orphan raised by the monks sets out on a journey. He meets many friends and each of them give him a souvenir stone. He is accompanied by an Ibex, who suggests that when he reaches the sea, he should throw all the stones into it. Isaac, with regret, agrees. However, joyful, he sees reflected in the water a beautiful colored mosaic of his figure, created by all the colorful stones. The Ibex tells him: "do you understand what the secret of our journey is?". "I think so" Isaac answered smiling.

"Every person we meet on our way" continued the Ibex "teaches us and gives us something. He or she gives us a more or less precious stone. If we know how to notice and keep these gifts in our hearts, we will become a small piece of who we met on the journey and who we met will become a very small piece of us. This is the secret!".

"Yes, that's right!" says Isaac smiling. "I will always remember the friends I met on this trip even if I won't see them again". It is an implicit reference to the meeting with the therapist.

Returning now to the dream, we see that the patient is paired with the analyst-notary, who summarizes the various segments of the experiences of separation that occurred in the temporal frame of reference of the past. There is also another possible couple with the hairdresser, who can allow the development of a conscious dialogue on the separateness to be conquered. In the associations there is first an attitude of frustration (later corrected) for the father's attitude that affects her impulsive oral behavior.

Finally, the associations end positively with an attitude of passionate dedication to the construction of the fairy tale. It is the expression of the temporary frame of reference of the present. It is precisely in this creativity that the patient captures the attitude of hope in continuing the self-analysis relating to the temporal frame of reference of the future. A progressive evolution emerged in the light of the MDAC criterion. A concluding therapeutic session was held. As in the other cases, the end of the analysis follows shortly.

Conclusions

In our opinion, the presented clinical cases prove that the proposed phenomenological criterion of the "concluding therapeutic turn" (CTT) is suitable for the purpose it pursues - to ascertain whether the patient has already achieved sufficient awareness of the path of change she has chosen. In the cases discussed, the patients showed that they could integrate their memories and emotions about significant problems of their past with a positive, constructive view of the present and a hopeful view of the future.

Etchegoyen, in a 1986 paper, reported very clearly on the various clinical signs that indicate the imminence of the completion of an analysis. He believed that the whole process needs a lot of time. The patient needs this time to arrive at an adequate mental representation of the hidden pathogenic text that she did not have before. Certainly, Etchegoyen correctly points out that a single indicator is not sufficient to complete the analysis. But if there are several such indicators and this in different contexts, it makes us think with confidence that we are on the right track.

On the problem of the conclusion of an analytic therapy, De Simone (1994) pointed out a crucial turning point for it, where the pending separation of the patient from her therapist is combined with the awareness of temporality, with a spotlight on the reality of temporal processes and the resulting reordering of psychic reality.

We think that the clinical understanding of therapy progressions can be expanded by adding to the various indicators already elaborated the criterion of the "concluding therapeutic turn" (CTT) presented in the present work. This is characterized by the connection and reconciliation with the three temporal reference systems while maintaining positive relational dynamics. Such a turn has for the patient all the characteristics of a psychic event that is new for her. Recognizing this is important not only for the patient, who is thus shown her therapeutic progress, but also for the analyst, in order to make this progress of his patient clearly visible to him.

We have seen that it is important to keep in mind both criteria, i.e., the MDAC criterion as well as the CTT criterion, in the session in order not to run the risk of drawing wrong conclusions. Here is an example of such a wrong conclusion:

A lady already advanced in her therapy had brought a dream in which she was to marry a friend from her music choir, a "choir in which one walks in harmony". The friend is a determined person who takes many initiatives: it is an aspect that the patient would like to integrate harmoniously into her own personality, to overcome her own lack of initiative from which she has always suffered. Initially, I (GT) thought it was a dream that connected the temporal frame of reference of the past with that of the present in relation to the patient's fundamental problem of making decisions. I had also noticed that in the temporal frame of reference of the present, to her own amazement, the patient had begun to take some initiatives in working with her husband. Thus, I was pleased and interested in the possibility that the session would be one of CTT. Unfortunately, this was not the case, as was shown in the associations towards the end of this session in the light of the MDAC criterion: this conclusion was negative, it consisted in an account of a recent example of her inability to bring to her husband's attention a cultural project that she wanted to carry out independently. It was not, therefore, a session of concluding therapeutic turn as discussed here. This was confirmed by the fact that the patient opened the next session with the words: "I dreamed of my other half. This is my cousin, a person crushed by her duties, knocking on my door." - the patient clearly expresses her conflict: the turning point still has to be reached.

Consideration of both the MDAC and CTT criteria can give the practitioner critical confidence in the maturation process of the therapeutic enterprise. In the therapeutic turn addressed here, there may also be agreement between the patient and the therapist about the termination of therapy. The CTT criterion helps the therapist recognize the right time to conclude the analysis. Recognizing this therapeutic turn also helps the analyst confront his patient's fear of living her new life without the support of the therapy sessions, as well as her sadness about the upcoming separation. The therapist knows at this point that the patient has developed sufficient awareness of her change. He can rightly comfort her in the hope that with the separation she will take another step toward solidifying her own identity.

10. Relational Determination in Interpersonal and Intrapsychic Experience

Edward S. Ragsdale [45]

Summary

This article reviews the principle of relational determination (RD) of meaning, as described by Solomon Asch (1952), which expands upon Karl Duncker's 1939 critique of ethical relativism. RD's conception of human conflict provides a path to understanding and even reconciliation of value differences – through cultivation of relational understanding. My goal is to extend its application of RD beyond the interpersonal/societal realm, to intrapsychic conflict, and particularly to the psychical polarization that underlies, and predisposes one to absolutist, dualist morality. This relational view opposes basic assumptions (e.g., elementarism, meaning constancy) common to both moral absolutism and relativism. Such assumptions lead to ill-considered conclusions: of irreconcilable moral differences dividing both individuals and groups, absent any basis in understanding. Those views fail to consider the contexts underlying the meanings and valuations we impute. When contexts and meanings are taken into account, Gestalt relationality (including at its core Duncker's 1939 hypothesis of a meaning-value invariance) finds support. Value differences (or changes) need not represent fundamental differences in morality, but instead (factual) differences in understanding of the situation. The potential for understanding and reconciliation that RD reveals in the case of interpersonal and societal conflict appears also to extend to intrapsychic conflict, which is burdened by the same absolutist, dualist presumption of irreconcilable differences. Work by Erich Neumann provides a depth psychological perspective on these Gestalt field-theoretic view. Neumann's depiction of a "new ethic" arising out of absolutism's growing dysfunction vividly illustrates the potential of relational understanding to heal inner divisions. The growth of awareness of contexts underlying conscious experience allows relational determination to manifest in relational understanding. In the process, intrapsychic realms of value, which earlier dwelt in hostile opposition, develop more respectful and communicative relation with each other, toward greater wholeness. Hopefully this relational viewpoint can be of service to Gestalt Theoretical Psychotherapy, in its efforts to ease conflict and increase understanding, not only in outer relations but in the crucible of inner experience as well.

Introduction

To me, a singular gift of Gestalt theory is its appreciation of a genuine capacity for insight and understanding in our species. Could there be a greater expression of that capacity than the formulation of a credible theory to support it? In my view, Gestalt theory's relational account provides such a foundation.

---

[45] This is a revised version of an article originally published in 2021 in a special issue of the e-journal *Gestalt Theory*, 43(1), 121-141; a German version appeared in the same year in the journal *Phänomenal*, 13(1), 11-27, under the title "Auf die Beziehung kommt es an. Relationale Determination im interpersonellen und intrapsychischen Erleben".

Its relational view sees experience taking shape as a function of relations and contexts. In the cognitive realm, it links insight and understanding to *awareness* of the relations giving rise to such experience. Gestalt theory's trust in a human faculty for truth and veridicality has set it apart from mainstream psychological schools (e.g., behaviorism, classical psychoanalysis) whose views are largely predicated on human blindness and self-interest. Besides calling into question the truth-value of their own pronouncements,[46] these reductionist accounts invite us to live down to the low level they set for our species (an invitation we hopefully do not accept). Gestalt theory's relational conception of human nature (and of order throughout nature), suggests we are capable of something more. I believe that Gestalt theory's field-theoretic, relational view helps to bring this into focus. In my eyes, that relational view remains a goldmine for further revelations, including our critical need to better understand and address the issues that divide us – both externally, in our relations with other persons and groups, and also internally, as regards intrapsychic conflict, which is clearly a focal concern of Gestalt Theoretical Psychotherapy.

Central to Gestalt theory is its *principle of relational determination*. As regards cognition (and certainly social cognition), we may speak of the relational determination of meaning and value. According to that principle, the meaning one imputes to an object of judgment (e.g., a particular practice or belief) depends upon the context in which one apprehends it. Likewise, the valuation one ascribes to it is deemed to follow fittingly from that (contextually-based) meaning. If so, then differences (or changes) in the object's valuation may reflect corresponding differences in the context that gives rise to that meaning. In that case, instances of value difference and value change need not reflect basic differences in morality, but instead differences in factual beliefs or understanding. This viewpoint allows for understandability in moral experience, in a moral universe that is big enough for all.

Plausible as it may appear, this Gestalt-theoretic view is at odds with viewpoints found at both ends of the familiar absolutism/relativism moral spectrum. Despite their polar opposition, both absolutism and relativism manage to agree as regards a quite important, though questionable proposition: In their shared disregard of the role of context and meaning in moral experience, they view value differences and value change to be as absolute and irreconcilable. True to its name, absolutism lays out categorial judgments, deemed to

---

[46] If indeed "science can have no more weight and sense than it itself attributes to the human insight by which it is produced" (Köhler 1938, 38).

apply universally across all contexts and situations. If meaning is considered at all, it is assumed to be fixed, and unaffected by changes in context. Here, a judgment or practice can (or should?) have no other meaning than that which supports the valuation it pronounces as absolute. Any departures from absolutism's rigidly dualistic view of goodness are simply deemed evil.

Next consider relativism, which is well prepared to accept fact of moral diversity, since it rejects the possibility of any overriding moral sensibility across humanity. Initially, it may have simply overlooked the possible role of meaning in moral judgments, at least until Karl Duncker's (1939) exposed relativism's implicit assumption of *"meaning constancy,"* (Duncker 1939, 47). Relativism's response (at least when it was being thorough) was to formally embrace that assumption. Thus, in all the cases of value conflict that relativists now offer in support of their position, it is presumed that persons who attach opposing valuations to a particular belief or practice nevertheless have in mind the same exact object of judgment (i.e., whose meaning is fixed despite opposing valuations). Where "change in meaning" is ruled out, variations in moral judgment can only be seen to reflect absolute and irreconcilable differences in morality – which, as such, can make no appeal to facts, beliefs, or understanding to try to reconcile *or even understand* their differences. This assumption of basic value differences, shared by both absolutism and relativism, would have us believe (largely in advance of investigation of a largely empirical question) that there are fundamental, presumably irreconcilable divisions cleaving humanity. Equally problematic, it would deprive moral experience any basis in reason or understanding – nor any basis for even considering questions of validity.

Gestalt theory, by way of its principle of relationality, offers another way of understanding value conflict – one that which makes room for the possibility of understandability (and potential reconcilability) of value differences throughout humanity, who may all have a home within the same moral universe. In their application of relational determination to the problem of interpersonal and inter-societal conflict, Gestalt theorists (e.g., Asch 1952; Duncker 1939) have greatly illuminated the problem of value conflict (whose accounts, given their vast implications, deserves much more attention than it has so far gotten.) That relational view encourages deeper examination of the contexts underlying differences in comprehension of the situation, for value differences may reflect such differences in meaning. Need to more closely examine underlying contexts applies not only to views with which we disagree, but also to the contexts supporting our own attitudes and values, which may not be as consciously accessible or well-differentiated as we would like to think (see Asch 1952, 367). As it turns out, imputations of absoluteness tend to preempt deeper inquiry into the grounds of value judgments, obscuring their relational basis beneath a veneer of absolutism. We will soon consider some structural features of the psychological situation which fuel resistance to deeper inquiry of the bases our own and others' competing views. Ironically, relational determination helps to make sense of our resistance to greater understanding (which is to say, our blindness to relational determination!).

The insights that the relationality principle offers as to interpersonal and societal conflict would seem to readily apply to problems of daily life that psychotherapists face every day in our work with clients. But from the goldmine that is relational determination, there is more to be mined. For human conflict is not confined to interpersonal intergroup situations. Most of us will agree from personal experience that there is no dearth of conflict on the intrapsychic front. Internal conflict appears to have the same structural properties as interpersonal and group conflict (as illustrated by GTP's use of "chairwork", or the "empty chair" (e.g., Stemberger 2014) as means of reducing conflict and increasing understanding between warring parts of self). Moreover, since the psychical system is likely organized, at least in part, around the need to manage (however imperfectly) internal conflict, the field-theoretic approach might well shed light on the organization of the psychical system generally. In the process, some further implications of relational determination come to light, and new aspects will be revealed in its application to some novel features of the intrapychic setting. Two concepts, *absolutization* and *polarization*, will hopefully be helpful in exploring these new arenas. Recognizing a need to distinguish my own theorizing from more established views of relational determination, I refer to these new applications of the relationality principle as the "Polarization Model" – it being one way in which relationality might conceivably manifest when applied to intrapsychic organization. One might question whether these speculations belong in a book laying out "essentials" of the GTP school of psychotherapy – which is a matter for time and our larger community to decide.

I admit that I am still getting acquainted with GTP, which is largely unknown in America (a problem the language barrier doesn't help). Of course, Gestalt theory has little active presence in America generally. I am thankful to GTA for connecting me with ongoing work. And I continue to find inspiration from earlier generations – including a second generation of American Gestaltists. Among them is Solomon Asch, a giant in American psychology, whose work, regrettably, is not well-known in Europe. When I think of the relational determination of meaning (and value), it is mainly Asch's view I have in mind (well-described in his 1952 masterwork *Social Psychology*). That account builds upon the earlier work of Karl Duncker. Duncker's 1939 critique of ethical

145

relativism put forth an extraordinary hypothesis – of an *invariant relation between meaning and value* – which is at the core of Asch's view of relational determination. This idea of an organic relation between the meanings (apprehended) and valuations (ascribed) opposes a core presumption of elementaristic psychology that was mentioned earlier – meaning constancy – which is a particularly problematic illustration of the *constancy hypothesis* that Gestalt theory took shape to oppose (Köhler 1947). Preemptive conclusions of irreconcilable differences follow inescapably from those elementaristic assumptions. Sadly, that same *appearance* of irreconcilability that often arises in our experience of external conflict may arise *within* the crucible of the human mind and heart. Let us see whether relational determination might offer as much to our understanding of intrapsychic conflict as it does to our understanding of interpersonal or cross-cultural differences.

In the course of discussion, I will explore other familiar GTP themes from the viewpoint of relational determination. Relational determination would seem to demand the use of *phenomenology* – not only as a starting point for science (Köhler 1947), but in the service of conscious development generally, since all conscious experience is grounded there. But while indispensable to human life, phenomenology is not an entirely reliable source of unvarnished truth. For naïve experience introduces some systematic distortions to its perception of the world. Gestalt theory employs *critical realism* (Stemberger 2021, Sternek 2021) to help identify and correct for blind spots and distortions of naïve perception. Obviously, a crucial part of perceptual experience – and for that matter, phenomenal experience generally – is the experiencing subject (who is also regularly an object of its own, self-conscious experience). What might relational determination have say as to the nature of the *"ego" and "self"* who are the subjects of experience (including experience of themselves experiencing). We may ask how well phenomenological experience, including experience of "I" and "me" aligns with relational understanding. Note here that relational determination cannot presume relational understanding. One's level of relational understanding seems bound to play a huge role in the character (indeed, the relational determination) of that experience. Mindful of that, we may ask how limitations in relational understanding of oneself (including the clients we seek to help) might affect one's experience of selfhood. We may also wonder how "I" or "me" might think or feel – or experience self and others – were that person fully awake to relational determination. In what follows, we will tread a path to these questions.

1. Relational Determination of Meaning and Value

So, our main topic is the *relational determination of meaning and value*, as described by Asch (1952) – at the heart of which is Duncker's (1939) hypothesis of an *invariant relation of meaning and value*. To repeat, relational determination boils down to the following: *The valuation of a thing (e.g., a belief, practice, or other object of judgment) is a function of the meaning that is imputed to it, which, similarly, is a function of the context in which it is understood.* In short (and in reverse order): Contexts give rise to meanings, and meanings give rise to valuations. Notice in this proposition Duncker's (1939) idea of an invariant relation between meaning and value – in that the valuation ascribed to an object of judgment (e.g., a belief or practice) is assumed to follow fittingly from its (context-dependent) meaning. Thus, any change or difference in valuation is predicted to involve a change in meaning (due to change in context).[47] This would preclude the possibility that two persons could interpret a given practice identically, yet disagree as to its valuation (which would deny reason any role in moral judgments) Relational determination rejects what Asch describes as the "essential proposition of ethical relativism" which states that "one can connect to the identical situation different and even opposed evaluations" (1952, 376).

An example may help to clarify the difference between Gestalt theory's relational view of relational determination and change-of-meaning, as opposed to relativism's assumption of absolute value differences and meaning constancy. Consider the heated conflict over abortion, which pits supporters of "right-to-life" against "pro-choice" advocates. Were this value conflict to be offered as evidence of relativism, the relativist would need to show that abortion has the same meaning for "right-to-life" believers as for "pro-choice" proponents.[48] Most, if not all, may find it hard to imagine that those in opposing camps, with opposing valuations, could possibly agree on what abortion means. Differences in meaning seem mainly to hinge upon different views as to the status of the fetus (at the time that abortion is considered). Right-to-lifers may view the fetus as a fully human being, and on that basis reject the practice as murderous. Pro-choice proponents may view abortion as the termination of a life form that is not yet fully human. The pro-choice attitude need not reject the idea that all humans have an equal right to life, but the applicability of that

---

[47] Note that the hypothesis of meaning-value invariance is not entirely reversable, since there could be changes in meaning that are not of a kind that would demand change in valuation.

[48] While conflicting attitudes toward abortion are most likely to turn on this issue, it should be noted that the value conflict could be linked to other factors besides the "personhood" or not of the fetus.

claim to the case of a perceived not-yet-human fetus (who has not yet achieved "personhood"). Attention may then shift to the rights of choice of the pregnant woman. In such cases, conflicting parties have no trouble identifying the "referent" of abortion, the practice to which the term refers. Yet in different contexts of belief, that same referent acquires quite different meanings and thus different valuations, which follow from one another in a fitting and understandable way. Thus, in contrast to meaning constancy, it we find (to paraphrase Duncker) that there are "two different meanings of [abortion], each of which receives its specific valuation" (1939, 41). Similarly, when valuations of an object change over time, Asch (1952) suggests that the change appears to be "in the object of judgment, rather than in the judgment of the object" (424).

But note here the important distinction between relational determination and *relational understanding* (a.k.a. insight). While Gestalt theory views all experience as relationally determined, that fact alone is no guarantee that the relational basis of experience will be recognized as such – either in specific cases, or as a general rule. There may or may not be the "direct awareness of determination" that Köhler calls "insight" (1947, 341),[49] and that Asch refers to as "relational understanding" (1952, 434). Relational understanding indicates *conscious awareness of the relations* that give rise to one's imputations of meaning and value. I find Asch's term useful because it reminds us of what insight or understanding is based on: awareness of underlying relations. Clearly there are times when relational awareness is obscured. At rare times, we may utterly blind to contexts, but they are generally at least partly in the reach of consciousness. I suspect they are rarely, if ever, fully complete. Lack of full awareness of relational determination – thus indicating some lack of relational understanding, indicates some lack of full access to the contexts that give rise the meaning one imputes. In those cases (which may represent the general case in human experience) relational determination is still assumed to apply, but to the extent one is blind to it, the determinative context (or some portion of it) may be considered implicit or unconscious. Such obscurations of understanding can also be viewed as reflections of limited conscious differentiation of the context or field. Thus full relational understanding would seem to entail a fully differentiated field.[50] Both characterizations – either in terms of implicit contexts or

---

[49] Elsewhere, in regard to the experience of requiredness or value, Köhler writes this (though he puts these words in the mouth of a perhaps rhetorical "editor"): "In recognizing the relations which make one thing demanded in a constellation of others, man exhibits what he calls *insight*" (Köhler 1938, 28).

[50] Note here that the conscious illumination of formerly implicit (or insufficiently differentiated) contexts exposes underlying beliefs or assumptions to reality-testing, which may cause some to be discarded or at least revised. The experience of fitting relations,

limited conscious differentiation – would appear to be interchangeable, since they are both describing the same thing in somewhat different ways. In sum, relational determination may manifest with varying degrees of relational understanding (depending upon individual acuity, the topic at hand, perhaps societal level of knowledge, etc.), and departures from full understanding are assumed to be indicative of limited conscious access to determinative contexts or, equivalently, to insufficient conscious differentiation of the field.

As regards the above example, it would seem that persons on both sides of the abortion issue have some ready access to a context of beliefs that lend support to their respective valuations. Despite this, the opposing camps remain at loggerheads. Their respective valuations are based on beliefs and assumptions the opposing party does not accept. As indicated above, a general problem regarding instances of value conflict, to be discussed later, concerns the often limited reach of relational understanding, which may have easy access to the immediate context, but less grasp of the relational basis of that context, and implicit contexts underlying it. After all, absolutist, dualist moralities can, perhaps always, find some basis in reason for their respective views, which may not be sufficiently penetrating to clarify the basis of all differences in factual belief. It is here that questions about establishing validity obtrude, which may be hard to answer without illuminating deeper strata of the relational field. Even if the thesis of relational determination is accepted, the task of achieving full relational understanding would seem mind-boggling. Such understanding is perhaps rarely if ever complete, though I see no *a priori* reason to rule out that potentiality (perhaps best exemplified in Buddhist views of enlightenment).

One other aspect of the relation between relational determination and relational understanding needs to be addressed, concerning the way that one's level of achievement of relational understanding is itself plays a role in the determination. That is, experience bears the effects of the presence of relational understanding, as well as its absence, and all points in between. More relationally informed states would seem to evince greater balance in their organization and less emotionality (cf. praegnanz?). Likewise, viewpoints with minimal relational understanding would appear to be somewhat less stable and more

---

connecting contexts to meanings to valuations, by no means guarantees the accuracy of underlying beliefs and assumptions, but it does point to the need to unearth these hidden contexts (or insufficiently differentiated fields) to be in a better position to assess the truth and generality of one's views.

emotionally reactive – as later discussion of "absolutization" will serve to illustrate.

2. Phenomenology

Clearly RD invites (indeed, requires) phenomenology – to help clarify the meanings underlying our valuations, and to illuminate the contexts that give rise to those meanings. Allow me to revisit Köhler's familiar observation that…

There seems to be a single starting point for psychology, exactly as for all other sciences: the world as we find it, naïvely and uncritically. The naïveté may be lost as we proceed. Problems may be found which were at first completely hidden from our eyes. For their solution it may be necessary to devise concepts which seem to have little contact with direct primary experience. Nevertheless, the whole development must begin with a naïve picture of the world. This origin is necessary because there is no other basis from which a science can arise. (Köhler 1947, 3)

This statement surely applies to the work of psychotherapy, not only because of its scientific aspect, but also because phenomenology is the basic modality of conscious life generally. A comment by Asch (1952) lingers in memory as a constant reminder:

"It...becomes clear that the first step in understanding action or conviction is to establish the way in which it appears to the actor and the reason it appears to him to be right." (Asch 1952, 381)

As Stemberger (2013, see also Böhm, 2021) notes about the psychotherapeutic relation – where the therapist seeks to understand the client, who seeks to understand herself – two phenomenal fields interact, each with its own phenomenology, with "theory of mind" active in both persons. (I recall from my years on the receiving end of therapy, how I often wanted to know how my therapist(s) perceived or responded to some specific situation in their lives, partly out of general interest, but also to better understand where they were "coming from" – with a vague sense of wanting to "triangulate," to have some additional point of reference about them to gain more perspective on them and on us.)

In any event, the client is challenged to faithfully describe her own actual experience. The therapist tries to absorb that communication with maximum fidelity to what is being shared (i.e., to respect her phenomenology). This is not to say that the therapist should not have, or make, judgments and interpretations, but that one needs to distinguish one's own beliefs and assumptions from the client's actual report, so as to reduce the risk of filtering the latter through the lens of the former. I find it daunting that my often overworked consciousness (and surely unconscious) is the lens (the emotional sense organ) upon which I must depend, to "know" the other. In that task, it surely helps to know oneself: The more I understand where I stop and my client begins – the less likely I am to conflate of the two realms. Of course I do not expect to reach full clarity and fidelity of perception anytime soon. This general human limitation illustrates a larger truth about experience in general: Whether we seek to honor only the "primary observational data" or accept any modifications that critical realism might bring to bear, experience may remain overlain with all manner of (often implicit) assumptions and predispositions – some universal, some enculturated, some distinctly idiosyncratic – which will continue shape experience in ways unbeknownst to the experiencer. Gestalt theory wisely draws attention to one widespread misapprehension – naïve realism – which is largely taken for granted across our species, even by those who "know" better.

3. Naïve Realism

Naïve realism errs in its failure to distinguish between the phenomenal and the physical object" (Henle 1977 in 1986, 3). It's "identification of percepts with physical things" (Köhler 1938, 405) takes the phenomenal (in this case, perceptual) experience to *be* the physical reality. Here phenomenology regularly misapprehends common *experience* of the world – mistaking it for unvarnished, subject-independent physical reality. We cannot conclude from this that relational determination fails to apply, but that experience may be far from fully cognizant of it. We see again, relational determination need not entail "relational understanding" (Asch 1952, 434). That is, perception (like phenomenal experience generally) need not *fully* possess the "direct awareness of determination" that Köhler (1947) describes as "insight" (341; see also 1938, 257).

Naïve realism's particular lack of relational understanding concerns its blindness as to the role of the sensory-perceptual system in the determination of perceptual experience. Absent that awareness, we construe the percept – which is in fact a product of interaction of distal/proximal input with the sensory-perceptual system – to constitute the unadulterated physical reality (which appears to be the sole cause of our experience of it). Thus, secondary qualities (e.g., color, taste, smell, sound) as well as tertiary qualities (which evoke emotional qualities (e.g. weeping willow, ominous clouds, bright disposition) – which arise as a function of this kind of subject-object interaction – instead appear to be real and self-evident properties of the physical entities themselves. This illustrates how a *lack* of relational understanding, here in regard to the role of the sensory/perceptual system, itself plays a role in the relational determination of the phenomenal experience (and by extension the associated physical entity), imbuing the percept with a sense of absolute, subject-independent existence.

4. Absolutization

This naïve attribution of independent (cf. absolute) existence to phenomenal entities may not be confined to the perceptual world. Naïve realism may be a subset of a more general pattern of misapprehension throughout phenomenal experience – reflecting its limited relational understanding. The problem concerns the consequences of any deficits of relational understanding as regards experience throughout the phenomenal world. To the extent we lack awareness of the relations that give rise to our conscious experience of meaning and value (or, put another way, to the extent that the contents of experience lack sufficient conscious differentiation to reveal their sheer relationality), those objects of experience will tacitly acquire a proportionate sense of *absoluteness* – such that they appear to be separate and independently existing entities, exhibiting qualities and characteristics that appear to arise from their own nature. Consider our routine attribution of absoluteness to the moral categories of good and evil. As was the case with naïve realism, blindness to relational determination may have a systematic effect one our experience of self and world – in imparting a sense of absoluteness to it. Below, Asch laments this general problem, identifies the nature of the effect, but offers no explanation.

"... It is hard to escape the conclusion that our naïve understanding of complex situations fails to take adequately into account their structured character and that we often endow social events with an *absoluteness* that is unwarranted.... Thinking, when it reaches the level of explicit self-awareness, may incline toward *absolutism* of method.... We shall not consider the reason for this shortcoming, but will attempt instead to show why we should think more resolutely in terms of relational determination if we are to do justice to social realities." (Asch 1952, 442-443, italics added)

Asch's comment, made in regard to social and political beliefs, would seem to apply generally across experience. It is perhaps reflected in our traditional predilection for absolutist morality (and for cognitive absolutism as well) – as a kind of *default-setting for experience short on relational understanding*. We are probably much less aware of the contexts that give rise to our own experience (i.e., the basis of our own imputations of meaning and value) than we would like to think [which Asch notes in the case of moral judgments (1952, 367-368)]. This may help to explain the absolutist form that all enculturated moralities appear to share. This is not to say that understanding is entirely lacking. One often has easy access to a body of credible facts and beliefs aimed at substantiating one's particular conception of the object of judgment. But it is likely harder to appreciate the relational basis of those contextual beliefs as well – the *context of that context*, as it were – which may be beyond our level of comprehension to grasp, or even to detect the lack of understanding. The greater the deficit of relational awareness, the stronger may be one's implicit (e.g., absolute) sense of truth of that context of supportive beliefs.

An explanation for this tendency to impute absoluteness to that which exists only relationally[51] may be hiding in plain sight. Here I am reminded of an article by Henle (1971/1986), which includes the quotation (by James Stephens) that "a well packed question carries its answer on its back as a snail carries its shell" (Stephens 1920, in Henle 1971/1986). As it turns out, the principle of relationality may itself hold the answer as to why it still dwells in relative obscurity. Assuming that experience is relationally determined, but is lacking in relational understanding, what recourse do we have but to attribute characteristics arising from (currently *unrecognized*) contextual relations, instead to the object of judgment itself – as though that object alone were the source of them? If one lacks awareness of the relations that give rise to particular qualities or attributes in the object, one is perhaps bound to attribute those characteristics to the object of judgment itself, as though they were intrinsic to it. The object may thus acquire a false or misleading appearance of absoluteness.

Köhler (e.g., 1947) and Asch (e.g., 1952) have described this as an object's "*assimilation*" of its context – which helps to explain some of the "face validity" of relativism in common experience. Here a valuation may attach itself "inseparably" to a behavior, with little regard to the situational meanings that originally generated it. That context may be so taken for granted, and thus so well ignored, that the associated valuation may be experienced as an inherent property of the behavior itself. When circumstances change, the conditions within which it maintained its former respect (which may have earlier gone unquestioned, and thus poorly articulated), grow even more remote. In the new context, the old behavior no longer fits. Absent memory of the credible context, the behavior itself may come to be faulted, as though it were wrong in and of itself, just as formerly it may have seemed right, in and of itself. Thus, we see how disregard of contexts and meanings may cause instances of value change to mistakenly appear to reflect absolute differences in values.

---

[51] Attentive readers may wonder if I am applying relational determination to the physical, as well as the phenomenal, world. Maybe? This was certainly the direction in which Köhler (1938) and other Gestalt psychologists were going.

I use the word *absolutization* to refer to the attribution, in varying degrees, of fixed, inherent meaning to objects and situations whose meaning is nevertheless relationally determined. Relational determination may thus serve not only to explain absolutization, but to predict it – as a natural consequence of a lack of relational understanding. In this case, the absolutization of experience masks its lack of relational understanding behind that false appearance of absoluteness. From this, we may conclude that relational determination can manifest in one of two ways (or in gradations in between): in either *relational understanding* or in *absolutization* (with the latter describing the form that ignorance is prone to take).

5. The Role of Motivations and Interests

Though absolutization may arise from what might be described as simple ignorance, there are at least *two* other factors that further fuel that blindness. The *first* concerns the effect of underlying motivations and conations. As Henle points out, a *"need or attitude may supply context"* (1949/1961 p.179). Up to now, we have looked at the contexts that give rise to meanings and valuations as cognitive fields. But value is not just something we take away from experience, it is also something we bring to it. Without some initial interest or motivation (including curiosity), objects need not even register in experience. The stronger the interest, the more determinative it may be in shaping experience of the object. Henle's observation thus seems not only accurate, but worthy of expansion: Conscious contexts perhaps invariably arise within motivated states, whose interests and agendas serve, *often tacitly*, to organize and direct the further differentiation of those contexts. Stemberger concurs, that the "[phenomenal] field is mainly organized by the needs and quasi-needs of the phenomenal ego on the one hand, and the attractive and repulsive properties in its phenomenal environment on the other" (Stemberger 2021, 5?)).

Note how underlying interests and motivations contribute to the appearance of meaning constancy: For example, when one is caught in desire or fear (cf. attraction or aversion), the object of interest may be sealed off within that affective field – to assume a meaning and valuation reflecting that interest alone (in that bubble, perhaps oblivious to other interests). Phenomenologically speaking, the force of attraction (or repulsion) will be felt to emanate directly from the phenomenal object (e.g., Köhler 1938). Attention likely focuses on the object instantiating the disposition, rather than the subjective state – which itself may draw little attention, given the force of its attraction to (or repulsion from) the object of interest. As was the case with cognitive contexts, to the extent the valuative field itself is disregarded, the object of interest at the center of that value field may acquire a *sense* of absolute good (or bad). Though its valuation is in fact *relative* to that value field, the intensity of that affective charge, together with one's obliviousness to other interests, may render that singular interest all-consuming (at least for as long as one remains under its spell). In extreme cases, the object may seem to exist only for the sake of the one perceiving it (as in the sexual objectification of one person by another).

This view suggests a new way of looking at cognitive and affective contexts (or fields), and the nature of their relation. An experiential context or field perhaps takes shape through (an ongoing) *cognitive articulation or differentiation of the affective/motivational field* whose interest is so engaged. That field is organized around the primary interest, likely to explore the means by which the object might be attained or avoided, etc.; or, if the affective charge leaves room for it, to survey the implications of pursuit or attainment of that object as regards other competing interests; Or seek to clarify the the understandable basis of one's interest; or, if that is fully clear, to simply to dwell in the sensations attendant to that interest (perhaps rapture, perhaps dread). Regardless of what is the case there, the main point here is that while *contexts give rise to valuations,* so too do *valuations (in this case, preexisting valuative dispositions) give rise to contexts.*

A *second* factor contributing to absolutization concerns the multiplicity of human interests and motivations, and their frequent lack of reconciliation – which is to say, their conflict. The most obvious aspect of the self, Henle suggests, may be the "... multiplicity of aspects it presents." (1962, p. 396). Some internal dialogues are well-aligned, as in Plato's description of thought as "the unuttered conversation of the soul with herself..." (in Henle 1962, 396). Other internal voices may impose themselves more pointedly – at times angrily, at other times supportively. As Montaigne observes, "we have a soul that can turn upon itself, that can keep company with itself; it has the wherewithal to attack and defend, to receive and give..." (Trechmann, trans, vol. 1, 238, in Henle 1962, 396).

Interests may instantiate in ways that align (in the same objects or goals), or in ways that conflict – patterns of affinity and conflict being somewhat specific to the person or the situation. The nature of these internal relations across different value states is evident in one's internal self-talk – at times attuned, at other times, impossibly discordant. For as Köhler notes, "in actual life, one requiredness is often the enemy of another..." (Köhler 1938, 210). It would seem that these different internal voices literally personify the particular value realm from which they arise, as well as the their attitudes towards one another. The element of personification is important, since it illustrates the role of personal identity as *agent* of the value realm with which one identifies. Just as objects of judgment acquire meanings that reflect the context in which they are understood, so too does self, or ego, assume an identity reflective of the value realm with which it currently identifies. That personal identity (i.e., the meaning that self acquires through identification with a context) represents the interests of that realm in unfolding experience. By attending to this internal messaging, and following it over time, one may arrive at some rough idea of the fault lines within the personality suggestive of its structural organization: the enforced boundaries (cf. defenses) dividing unreconciled realms; the level of differentiation within those realms; the nature of the relation, and quality of communication within and between realms, etc. Many will agree that one's internal dialogues may be even more belligerent than one's relations with human antagonists in the world outside. But throughout the "civilized" world, there is one intrapsychic demarcation common to all enculturated persons: The phenomenal worlds of each of us is divided in two by a moral battleline, evincing the lack of reconciliation between contrasting realms of value.

6. Polarization

The most common example of intrapsychic division, and probably the most consequential, concerns the conflict between the person's socially aligned interests, in the face of narrower interests whose satisfaction comes at the expense of the society. Out of that conflict, whose individual and societal implications are immense, formal morality likely emerged (when expanding and complexifying societies came to require a more concrete explication of their previously implicit sense of connection and care). This codification (whose enshrinement in a religious narrative helped to convey its transcendental authority) was elevated above all other value realms to become a standard for judging them – a development that may have given birth to formal morality. Note the exclusionary nature of absolutism, which entails dualism. One's embrace of accepted beliefs and values is likewise a repudiation of conflicting interests and proclivities. Rejected contents may unite as common objects of scorn, to form an opposing realm of absolute rejection. I use the word *polarization* to describe the morally differentiated psychical structure, organized around co-arising, yet opposing, part-contexts, which reflect the conflicting value realms (cf. motivations) on the basis of which each took shape. Early societal morality surely required such polarization, which pits good against evil in a simple and direct way, as the most reliable means of establishing moral restraint, and of maintaining the capacity for morally differentiation needed to exercise it.

Observe how polarization further heightens absolutization. One clings ever more tightly to absolute goodness, not just for its own sake, but also to resist darker attractions. This absolutization of value differences intensifies the absolutization of each realm, in part through a moral contrast effect: As the light seeks to become lighter, the dark grows darker and more vile.[52] Mere association with one realm or another may trigger preemptive judgment – stirring either credulous embrace or contempt prior to investigation, as opposed to open-minded reflection. While this moral sensibility may be well-motivated, it is mixed with other concerns – including the need for social acceptance, which absolutist morality has made conditional – upon fidelity to its morality, and/or public demonstration of it.

Consider moral polarization through the lens of relational determination. It begins with differentiation of a psychical whole on expressly moral lines. Individuals come to identify with one realm and dis-identify with the other. Each opposing realm (and identity) is defined in terms of the other – in this case as something the other is *not*. The two countenance no relation besides categorical opposition. This enforced separation of realms preempts any growth of understanding as might reveal commonalities, which might mitigate their opposing stance. This highly selective awareness (and bias) appears to be structural property of the polarized order – which elevates moral differentiation over other concerns. Any relaxation of categorical opposition may endanger this dualistic moral order, upon which further psychological and societal development may depend. However, maintenance of moral differentiation on the normative front may come at the cost of misconstruing the nature of moral differences on the epistemological (and perhaps ontological) front. Thus, relational facts come to appear absolute, I suggest that this is due to limited awareness of that relational basis, which leads to absolutization; as well as the blinding effect of the affective field in which such experience presents; and an effective redoubling of that affective charge due to polarization: In effect, one absolute is needed to battle another in this polarized force-field.

7. A Field-Theoretic View of Depth Psychology

At the risk of misplaced "eclecticism" (cf. Henle 1957/1986), allow me to introduce a depth psychological perspective – specifically Eric Neumann's Jung-inspired theory of societal moral development, which aligns surprisingly well with Asch's relational view. Neumann describes a time of *primal unity* in early human groups, which initially cohered around an implicit sense of connection and care. But as societies grew in size and complexity, the need grew for more explicit and codified morality. Thus emerged traditional absolutist morality, which Neumann calls "old ethic." I have retained Neumann's Jungian terminology – "persona" and "shadow" – to identify the old ethic's opposing

---

[52] Is it possible that the establishment of societal morality – especially in its rigidly dualistic form – has helped to fuel humanity's imagination for evil?

identities. It's rigid dualism presses members (in their familiar persona-identification) to renounce shadow aspects – which entails either *suppression* or *repression*. Those who can admit to their darkness must suppress and suffer it, while others, oblivious or in denial, rely more on repression and projection (i.e., externalization). Both adaptations (especially repression) lead to externalization of unacceptable contents onto familiar scapegoats – i.e., aliens, minorities, persons ill-equipped for moral adaptation (cf. criminals), also those who surpass the shared morality, and expose its insufficiencies. Absolutist morality inculcates morally differentiated consciousness (which was likely crucial to further human development). But its monumental success has come at the price of systematic distortions of experience, which over time render the morality susceptible to corruption, erosion, and cooptation. Neumann's rich account of this dysfunctionality never seems out of step with Asch's brief characterization. Despite their different theoretical perspectives, the general correspondence of their views provides an opportunity for cross-fertilization of ideas, not only regarding the structural problems of absolutism, but also their prescriptions for a remedy.

Regarding problematic aspects, consider the psychological defenses that Neumann finds endemic to absolutist morality. From the point of view of RD, these defensive operations may be seen as structural characteristics of polarized psychical organizations, whose moral order may be threatened by greater understanding. Consider the boundary between persona and shadow, which must be defended to preserve persona's moral integrity. From a field-theoretic point of view, this may involve a "sharpening" of boundaries between opposing value realms, and a "leveling" (or softening or blurring) of boundaries within respective value realms. One thus exaggerates differences between opposing realms, while minimizing differences within realms (particularly that of persona). The persona-realm thus presses for seamless unity of self, society, and the morality that connects them. This unification within provides security and fortification against the shadow without. These field-processes also manifest in one's experience of similarity and difference (cf. the attraction-similarity correlation). Within value realms, relations are organized around similarities, while between value realms relations are organized around differences.

Field-theoretic thinking also helps to illuminate the dynamics of repression and externalization (cf. projection). If we heed critical realism's reminder that what we take to be the physical world is actually a phenomenal representation of it, we can see more clearly that "projection" is not some operation upon a physical entity (e.g., another person) in the "real" world. What I prefer to call *externalization* takes place entirely within one's own phenomenal field – perhaps involving nothing more than a small shift in phenomenal boundary, or relocation of a content to the other side of it. This structural feature of the phenomenal field, which plays a part in its larger organization, exists independently of persons who may be phenomenally represented there, though it may be decisive in the way we view them. Our judgment of others is not just a reflection of them, but of us as well. In fact, our judgments of others may say more about ourselves than about the other. The quality of one's judgments reflects the quality of the organization of the phenomenal field of the one passing judgment – whether for example the phenomenal representation of oneself is sufficiently differentiated to bear awareness of personal imperfection within its own self-boundary, or whether any such imperfection must be represented outside that personal boundary, in a region of the field in which other persons or groups are phenomenally represented (in which case, anyone represented there, by that fact alone, would be imbued with some absolutized sense of villainy. Relational determination helps us to see that everything we experience is a part of ourselves, including our judgments of others.

Notice also the limitations of suppression as a moral adaptation. Imagine persons whose experiential field are sufficiently differentiated to "own" their personal imperfection. If, in that superior state of consciousness, they still view their culpability in absolutist terms, as something as utterly irreconcilable with the acceptable world, they may remain stuck in that impasse, with no means of cleanse themselves of moral stain. Without some amendment to its view, absolutism's way of establishing awareness of (moral) differences – as absolute and categorical moral differences – would deny persons a means to resolve them.

Not only do Neumann and Asch suggest antidotes to the blindness of absolutist morality. What they each propose appears to be the same cure, couched in different language. Both agree as to the insufficiency of absolutist morality. Both encourage growth of understanding that permits the reconciliation of differences, which absolutism (like relativism) views as irreconcilable. Consider Neumann's remedy: With some urgency, he presses for a reorientation of understanding toward a "new ethic," daring us to "'work through' our evil in an independent and responsible way."

The main function of the new ethic is to bring about a process of integration, and its first aim is to make the dissociated elements, which are hostile to the individual's program for living, capable of integration. The juxtaposition of opposites which makes up the totality of the world of experience can no longer be resolved by the victory of one side and the suppression of the other, but only a synthesis of these opposites. (Neumann 1969/1990, 101)

Neumann describes what this entails:

"If, instead of suppressing and repressing the contents of the unconscious, the new ethic is to "accept" them and articulate them with the conscious mind, it will inevitably be faced with the task of their assimilation.... In this process, contents which were previously split-off and autonomous are joined up to form parts of a comprehensive psychic structure which is connected with the ego and the conscious mind, and so *receive a different meaning and value* in the hierarchy." (p. 99, italics added)

The insights of Gestalt theory, upon which Gestalt Theoretical Psychotherapy draws, are tailor-made for this work – which is the work of growing consciousness. Its relational view appears invaluable in laying out a "royal road" to greater consciousness, through cultivation of relational understanding. Moral absolutism (with its inevitable dualism) has been indispensable in establishing moral consciousness, which apparently must depend upon moral polarization (thus absolutism and dualism) to institutionalize it, whose growing dysfunction is becoming too great to bear. The current challenge is not just to maintain moral consciousness, but to deepen it – by shedding reliance upon polarization to sustain it. This requires something like peace talks between warring factions of the self. There is perhaps no better illustration of this challenge than that found in a familiar therapeutic tool of GTP – involving "work with the empty chair" (e.g., Stemberger 2014). The exercise both conveys its emotional challenge and captures the essence of the theoretical view. Here one comes face-to-face with one's inner opposite – perhaps initially recoiling in bewilderment and disgust – often to discover mutual understanding, and even compassion and respect if that relation is allowed to unfold. Neumann suggests that we may have a moral duty face ourselves in this way (and thus spare others the burden of serving as our "projection" screen). It probably takes field theory to grasp the transformations involved in such psychological processes – where change in relation leads to changes the meaning and value of each participant in relation. In the process, one may come to outgrow polarization, while not only retaining moral consciousness but expanding it. Both Gestalt theory and Gestalt Theoretical Psychotherapy are well-positioned to support this further growth of consciousness – in part for the faith and trust they maintain in human understanding.

8. Critical Realism

The task of critical realism, as I see it, is to recognize and correct for any ways in which naïve experience distorts or blindly superimposes onto the percept, things that are not present in the actual physical reality. Naïve realism misconstrues perceptual experience through a particular failure of relational understanding (which in this case overlooks the role sensory/perceptual processes in the relational determination of experience). In my view, the easy part of critical realism is the mere recognition that the perceptual event (being a product in part of those sensory/perceptual processes) is not in itself the physical reality (see Sternek 2021, also in the current volume). But naïve realism's misconstrual may involve more than simple conflation of phenomenal and physical worlds. Any lack of awareness of relational determination (including that specific to naïve realism) may entail some reification or absolutization of experience (proportionate to the extent of relational blindness). Even when one can distinguish phenomenal and physical "reality," persons may continue to impute some sense of absolute existence (independent of context, experiencer, etc.) to things that exist only relationally.

This problem is not limited to perceptual experience but exists throughout the phenomenal world. Further analysis of that world may be needed, akin to what critical realism applies to naïve perceptual experience. As adherents to Gestalt theory, one standard we may be willing to apply is relational determination, which is presumed to apply throughout experience. Earlier I introduced the term *absolutization* to indicate a false or misleading attribution of absoluteness to experience that (assuming relationality applies) exists only relationally. Relational determination is not negated by any lack of awareness of it. But where relational understanding is at all lacking, those relational aspects may well be attributed, if only by default, to the object of judgment alone, as though they were inherent in it. Here the lack of relational understanding is masked by a blind imputation of absoluteness to the phenomenal object. This does not mean that persons with different degrees of relational understanding cannot meaningfully communicate about phenomenal or physical things. But it is unclear what epistemological (or ontological) status to assign phenomenal objects when their meaning (and even their existence) is understood to be a function of context in which it happens to be a *part*, especially when the variability of those context effects may be endless. When the larger context remains unspecified, and is subject perhaps to infinite variability, what kind of reality can be credibly assigned to an apparent entity, in and of itself, when its meaning is recognized to vary widely, based upon the context (explicit or implicit) in which it is apprehended. While in states of limited relational understanding, where some absolutization of experience can be expected, what epistemological (or ontological?) status might critical realism attach to an objects of judgment – given the contingencies that relational determination entails. Perhaps the critical question is how would that phenomenal entity appear – and what epistemological status could it rightly claim – in the full light of relational understanding.

9. "Ego" and "Self" in Phenomenological Experience and Theory

The preceding discussion is in great need of an example. This final topic, concerning the experience and factual basis of selfhood, happily provides one. And is all the better that we can begin with a comment by Wertheimer (as quoted by Stemberger in this current volume, whose fascination with this subject I share):

"Here I am – the ego – first a part of the field. I am not fundamentally an Ego standing in relief against other Egos, as has usually been maintained; no, the genesis of an Ego is one of the strangest and most remarkable of phenomena which, it would appear, is also controlled by whole-processes. As I have stated, I am part of this field." (Wertheimer 1924 in 1944, 90)

It is hard for me to understand the way in which I exist, since the "I" that I claim to be is not, and will never be, a free-standing entity, perhaps especially at times when I believe I am. In much the same way that my naïve realism mistakes the perceptual representations for the physical reality, I take a particular image of myself to constitute my actual being. But that ego-identity is not only a part of a larger whole, which itself keeps changing. It is hard to establish any final circumference to the contextual field that gives rise to me, or perhaps any other conscious being, nor to begin to fathom the subtleties of even the internal part-context which serves to phenomenally represent my "self" in its myriad states and identities. (While I know the phenomenal representation of myself cannot possibly be or coincide with my actual self, something needs to stand up and be counted, and it is surely the best that I've got.). Of course I am still routinely taken in by the self-image which mistake for reality – particularly when that image is under threat, or caught in self-aggrandizement. But it is pretty clear to me when I think about it, it's not quite "me" (whatever that could be). The experience of self that arises in bifurcated psychical structures – identifying with one realm, and occasionally its more questionable twin – must be glaringly misinformed, so entrenched in maintenance of an identity that rejects the very context that gives rise to it. Self-experience – at least where it clings to a particular image or impression, against inner doubt or outer besmirchment – relies upon defensive operations, which preserve not the actual self, nor a mere construct, but, in part, a practiced deceit. Gestalt theory helps to reveal these defensive operations as artifacts of particular psychical structure – a structure that thankfully is capable of further reorganization – through processes of further differentiation and further reconciliation of differences. Perhaps the more that relational understanding grows in the person, the more whole that person becomes, and the less conceptualizable that wholeness will be, in the freedom and comfort being a *part* of everything it meets.

Postscript:

Another article in this work (Zuczkowski & Stemberger 2022) serves to illustrate a number of topics discussed here, including   absolutization – all in regard to the problem of "feeling-causality." This is illustrated by an early experience of one of the authors, who, in bygone days, found himself blaming his wife for the anger she triggered in him – as though he was her innocent victim. [I am dispensing here with gender-neutrality (and for that matter, anonymity), since in this personal vignette, the author has already "outed" his central characters.] His therapist at the time reminded him of his ultimate responsibility for his reactions, which he soon recognized, but the episode continued to puzzle him: How and why in common experience do we so often view others as the "makers of our feelings." Gestalt theory's field-theoretic approach seems uniquely qualified to address this question – by applying some of its central concepts and methods (e.g., phenomenology, naïve realism, critical realism, relational determination, and perhaps even absolutization). *Phenomenology* might shed light on the understandable basis for his reaction, by taking a closer look at unfolding experience, which may have been compromised by some *naïve realm* on his part, in overlooking his own (interactive) role in its *relational determination* – a blind spot that *critical realism* helps to reveal. This limitation in *relational understanding,*(e.g., his blindness as to his own part in it, perhaps led to the *absolutization* of his wife's alleged provocation, prompting his reactive anger. Consider now the therapist's suggestion that he consider himself the cause of his own reactions. One way of operationalizing that view is to re-imagine the entire episode unfolding, not in the physical world, but in his own phenomenal field, which is the only realm we have in which to know self and world. And to remember that one's manner of being in the world reflects one's experience of relations across phenomenal field, corresponding to the relations we have with actual people we know. One way of taking responsibility for our own behavior is to remember that we ourselves are overseers of that entire phenomenal field, with the opportunity to bring as much consciousness as we can into that experience, so as to maximize our understanding of self and other, regardless of what that other does or does not do. The greater our level of relational understanding, the less prone we are to relatively blind, emotional reactivity.

Bibliography

Agazarian, Yvonne M. (1986): Application of Lewin's life space concept to the individual and group-as-a-whole systems in psychotherapy. In E. Stivers & S. Wheelan (Eds.), *The Lewin legacy: Field theory in current practice*. New York: Springer-Verlag, 101–112.

Agazarian, Y. M. (2004): *System-Centered Therapy for Groups*. New York, Routledge.

Andersch, Norbert (2012): Hans Carl Leuners Monographie: 'Die experimentelle Psychose' und sein Konzept einer 'konditional-genetischen Psychopathologie'. In B. Holdorff & E. Kumbier (Hrsg.), *Schriftenreihe der Deutschen Gesellschaft für Geschichte der Nervenheilkunde DGGN, Band 18*, 197–212.

Andersch, N. (2014): *Symbolische Form und psychische Erkrankung. Argumente für eine ,Neue Psychopathologie'. Klinische und philosophische Überlegungen*. Würzburg: Königshausen & Neumann.

Andersch, N. & John Cutting (2014): Ernst Cassirer's Philosophy of Symbolic Forms and its impact on the theory of psychopathology. *History of Psychiatry, 25*(2), 1–21.

Arfelli Galli, Anna (2012): *Gestaltpsychologie und Kinderforschung*. Wien: Krammer.

Asch, Solomon E. (1952): *Social psychology*. Englewood Cliffs, NJ: Prentice Hall.

Asch, S.E. (1958): Cacophonophobia. Review of Festinger, A Theory of Cognitive Dissonance. *Contemporary Psychology, 3*, 194–195.

Ash, Mitchell G. (1995): *Gestalt Psychology in German Culture 1890–1967. Holism and the Quest for Objectivity*. Cambridge University Press.

Balsamo, Maurizio (2019): *Ascoltare il presente*. Milano: Mimesis.

Bandler, Richard & John Grinder (1975): *The structure of magic*. Palo Alto: Science and Behavior Books.

Baranger, Madeleine & Willy Baranger (2008/1961): The analytic situation as dynamic field. *The International Journal of Psychoanalysis, 89*, 795–826.

Barwinski, Rosmarie (2014): Die therapeutische Beziehung. *Psychotherapie-Wissenschaft, 4*(1), 2–3.

Beckmann, Jürgen & Heinz Heckhausen (2018): Situational Determinants of Behavior. In Heckhausen, J. & H. Heckhausen (Eds.), *Motivation and Action*, 3rd edition, Springer, 113–162.

Becvar, Dorothy S. (2003): Eras of epistemology: A survey of family therapy thinking and theorizing. In: Sexton, T. L., G. R. Weeks, M.S. Robbins (Eds.), *Handbook of family therapy*. New York and Hove: Brunner-Routledge, 3 – 20.

Beneder, D. (2015): Gestalttheorie und Diagnostik in der Psychotherapie – Eine kommentierte Auswahlbibliographie. *Phänomenal, 7*(2), 51–55.

Beneder, Doris (2011): „ICD 10-Diagnose? Das mache ich doch nur für die Kasse!" *Phänomenal, 3*(1), 3–7.

Berne, E. (1964): *Games people play*. New York: Grove Press.

Berne, E. (1972): *What do You Say after You Say Hello?* Beverly Hills: City National Bank.

Berne, Eric (1961): *Transactional Analysis in Psychotherapy*. New York: Grove Press.

Bezoari Michele & Antonino Ferro (1992): Il sogno all'interno di una teoria del campo: aggregati funzionali e narrazioni. In: Eugenio Gaburri (a cura di, 1997), *Emozione e interpretazione*. Torino: Bollati Borlinghieri.

Bigi, Arrigo (2004): La capacità di finire l'analisi. *Rivista di Psychoanalisi*, 3, 639-663.

Bischof, Norbert (1966): Erkenntnistheoretische Grundlagenprobleme der Wahrnehmungspsychologie. In W. Metzger & H. Erke (Hrsg.), *Handbuch der Psychologie in 12 Bdn. Bd. 1/I: Wahrnehmung und Bewusstsein*. Göttingen: Verlag für Psychologie, 21-78.

Bischof, Norbert (2014): *Psychologie. Ein Grundkurs für Anspruchsvolle*. 3. Auflage. Stuttgart: Kohlhammer.

Blum, Harold P. (2011): Sogni rivisitati. *Rivista di Psychoanalisi*, 2, 385-388.

Boothe, B.; Becker-Fischer, M. & G. Fischer (1993): Die ‚ewige Tochter': Ein neuer Ansatz zur Konfliktpathologie der magersüchtigen Frau. In G.H. Seidler (Hg.): *Magersucht. Öffentliches Geheimnis*. Vandenhoeck & Ruprecht: Göttingen, 87-133.

Böhm, Angelika (2011): Phänomenale Kausalität: Ein gestalttheoretischer Beitrag zur Wirkungsforschung. *Phänomenal, 3*(1), 34-39.

Böhm, A. & G. Stemberger (2018): Gestalttheoretische Psychotherapie. In: M. Hochgerner (Hrsg.), *Grundlagen der Psychotherapie. Lehrbuch zum Psychotherapeutischen Propädeutikum*. Wien: facultas, 181–191.

Böhm, A. (2021): Basic Principles for Therapeutic Relationship and Practice in Gestalt Theoretical Psychotherapy. *Gestalt Theory, 43*(1), 69-86.

Böhm, A. (2022): Basic Principles for Therapeutic Relationship and Practice in Gestalt Theoretical Psychotherapy. Revised version of Böhm 2021. *Current volume.*

Bolognini, Stefano (2008): *Passaggi segreti*. Torino: Bollati Borlinghieri.

Bozzi, Paolo (1969): *Unità, Identità, Causalità*. Bologna: Cappelli.

Brown, Junius F. (1929): The methods of Kurt Lewin in the psychology of action and affection. *Psychological Review*, 36, 200–221.

Brown, J. F. (1933): Über die dynamischen Eigenschaften der Realitäts- und Irrealitätsschichten. *Psychologische Forschung, 18*(1/2), 2-26.

Bruch, Hilde (1962): Perceptual and Conceptual Disturbances in Anorexia Nervosa. *Psychosomatic Medicine, 24*(2), 187-194.

Bruch, H. (2000): *Der goldene Käfig. Das Rätsel der Magersucht*. Frankfurt am Main: Fischer.

Buchholz, Michael B. & M. Dümpelmann (1993): Väter bei Anorexie. In G.H. Seidler (Hg.): *Magersucht. Öffentliches Geheimnis*. Vandenhoeck & Ruprecht: Göttingen, 53-86.

Buchholz, Michael B. (2020): Seeing the situational Gestalt. Movement in therapeutic spaces. *Gestalt Theory, 42*(2), 101-132.

Buchmann, Rudolf; Schlegel, Mario; Vetter, Josef (1996): Die Eigenständigkeit der Psychotherapie in Wissenschaft und Praxis. In: Pritz, A. (Hrsg.), *Psychotherapie – eine neue Wissenschaft vom Menschen*. Wien: Springer, 75-122.

Cali, Carmelo (2007): Isomorphism and mirror neuron system. Commentary Article on Eagle M. N. & Wakefield J. C., Gestalt Psychology and the Mirror Neuron Discovery. *Gestalt Theory 29*(2),168-173.

Canestrari, Renzo & Giancarlo Trombini (1975, 2019): Psychotherapie als Umstrukturierung des Feldes. In: Ertel, Kemmler & Stadler (Hrsg., 1975), *Gestalttheorie in der modernen Psychologie*, Darmstadt: Steinkopff, 266-273. Reprinted in a revised version in 2019: *Phänomenal, 11*(2), 29-35.

Carloni, Glauco (1991): Il sogno nella pratica psicoanalitica di oggidi'. In: Marino Bosinelli & PierCarla Cicogna (a cura di): *Sogni: figli di un cervello ozioso*. Torini: Bollati Boringhieri.

Cash, Thomas F. & Edwin A. Deagle 3rd (1997): The nature and extent of body-image disturbances in anorexia nervosa and bulimia nervosa: a meta analysis. *International Journal of Eating Disorders, 22*, 107-125.

Clark, Andy (2012): Embodied, embedded, and extended cognition. In: Frankish, K. & RW. M. Ramsey (Eds.), *The Cambridge handbook of cognitive science*. Cambridge: Cambridge University Press, 275-291.

Corr, Philip J. & Gerald Matthews (Eds., 2009): *The Cambridge handbook of personality psychology*. Cambridge, UK: Cambridge University Press.

Corsini, Raymond J. & Danny Wedding (2010): *Current Psychotherapies* (9th Edn). Belmont, CA: Brooks/Cole.

De Rivera, Joseph (1976): *Field Theory as Human Science. Contributions of Lewin's Berlin Group*. New York: Gardner Press.

De Simone, Gilda (1994): *La conclusione dell'analisi*. Roma: Borla.

De Toffoli, Carla (2008): Funzione evolutiva dei fenomeni di transfert. In: Anna Ferruta (a cura di), *I transfert. Cambiamenti nella pratica clinica*. Roma: Borla, 35-44.

Dembo, Tamara (1931 in 1976): The Dynamics of Anger. (Translation of Dembo 1931, Der Ärger als dynamisches Problem, by Hedda Korsch). In: De Rivera 1976, 324–422.

Di Chiara, Giuseppe (2003): *Curare con la psicoanalisi*. Milano: Cortina.

Dilling, H. & H.J. Freyberger (2016, Hrsg.): *ICD 10*. Göttingen: Hogrefe.

Duch, Wlodzislaw (2018): Kurt Lewin, psychological constructs and sources of brain cognitive activity. *Polskie Forum Psychologiczne, 23*(1), 7-21.

Duncker, K. (1939): Ethical relativity? (An enquiry into the psychology of ethics). *Mind, 48*, 39-57.

Duncker, Karl (1935): *Zur Psychologie des produktiven Denkens*. Berlin: Springer.

Eagle, Morris N. & Jerome C. Wakefield (2007): Action Potentials and Representationality: Reply to Dr. Cali's Commentary. *Gestalt Theory, 29*(2), 173-175.

Eliot, T.S. (1959): *The Elder Statesman*. London, UK: Faber and Faber.

Etchegoyen, R. Horacio (1986): *Los Fundamentos de la Tecnica Psicoanalitica*. Buenos Aires: Amorrortu Editores.

Falci, Amedeo (2005): Sulla definizione di fattori aspecifici nella terapia psicoanalitica. In: Giuseppe Berti Ceroni (a cura di), *Come cura la psicoanalisi*. Milano: Franco Angeli, 157-171.

Ferro, Antonino (1999/2003): *The Bi-Personal Field: Experiences of Child Analysis*. London & New York: Routledge 1999. *Das bipersonale Feld. Konstruktivismus und Feldtheorie in der Kinderanalyse*. Gießen: Psychosozial Verlag 2003.

Festinger, Leon (1957): *A Theory of Cognitive Dissonance*. Evanston, Ill.: Row, Peterson.

Flückiger, Christoph; Horvath, Adam O.; Del Re, A.C., Symonds, Dianne & Corinne Holzer (2015): Bedeutung der Arbeitsallianz in der Psychotherapie. Übersicht aktueller Metaanalysen. *Psychotherapeut, 60*(3), 187–192.

Foschi, Renato & Giovanni P. Lombardo (2006): Lewinian contribution to the study of personality as the alternative to the mainstream of personality psychology in the 20th century. In J. Trempata et al. (Eds.), *Lewinian Psychology. Proceedings of the*

International Conference „Kurt Lewin: Contribution to Contemporary Psychology". Bydgoszcz, Poland: Kazimierz Wielky University Press, 86–98.

Fuchs, Thomas (2010): „Ich weiß, wie dünn ich bin, aber ich fühle mich dick". Gestalttheoretisches Modell der wahrgenommenen Welt einer magersüchtigen Person. *Phänomenal, 2*(2), 3–9.

Fuchs, Th. (2014): Die praktische Seite einer Erkenntnistheorie: Zur Entwicklung einer angemessenen therapeutischen Haltung in der Arbeit mit essgestörten Menschen. *Gestalt Theory, 36*(2), 129-140.

Fuchs, Th. & G. Stemberger (2018): Über das Hinzuziehen weiterer Personen zur Psychotherapie. *Phänomenal, 10*(1), 38-42.

Fuchs, Th. (2020): Vom Miteinander, Gegeneinander und Nebeneinander in der Therapie. *Phänomenal, 12*(2), 17-26.

Fuchs, Th. (2021): Gestalt Theoretical Psychotherapy – A Clinical Example. *Gestalt Theory, 43*(1), 87-99.

Fuchs, Th. (2022): Gestalt Theoretical Psychotherapy – A Clinical Example. Reprint of Fuchs 2021. *Current volume.*

Galli, Giuseppe (1997 in 2017): Beziehungen zwischen Lewins wissenschaftstheoretischen Begriffen und der Psychoanalyse. *Gestalt Theory, 19*(2/1997), 80-89. Reprint in Galli 2017, 107–115.

Galli, G. (1999): *Psychologie der sozialen Tugenden.* Wien: Böhlau.

Galli, G. (2005): *Psychologie der sozialen Tugenden.* Zweite, erweiterte Auflage. Wien: Böhlau.

Galli, G. (2010, Hrsg.): *Gestaltpsychologie und Person. Entwicklungen der Gestaltpsychologie.* Wien: Krammer.

Galli, G. & G. Trombini (2013): Das Problem des Bezugssystems in der Psychotherapie. *Phänomenal, 5*(1-2), 19-22. Also in Galli 2017, 116-123 (Die Theorie des Bezugssystems und ihre Anwendung in der klinischen Situation).

Galli, G. (2017): *Der Mensch als Mit-Mensch. Aufsätze zur Gestalttheorie in Forschung, Anwendung und Dialog. Herausgegeben und eingeleitet von Gerhard Stemberger.* Wien: Krammer.

Goulding, M.M. & R.L. Goulding (1979): *Changing Lives through Redecision Therapy.* New York: Brunner and Mazel.

Goulding, Mary M. & Robert L. Goulding (1978): *The Power is in the Patient.* San Francisco: TA Press.

Graefe, Oskar (1961): Über Notwendigkeit und Möglichkeit der psychologischen Wahrnehmungslehre. *Psychologische Forschung, 26,* 262–298.

Hall, Calvin S. & Gardner Lindzey (1978): *Theories of personality* (3rd ed.). Hoboken, NJ: John Wiley & Sons.

Harrington, Ann (1996): *Reenchanted Science. Holism in German Culture from Wilhelm II. to Hitler.* Princeton University Press.

Harrower, Molly (1983): *Kurt Koffka – An Unwitting Self-Portrait.* Gainesville: University Presses of Florida.

Heckhausen, Heinz (1991): *Motivation and Action.* Berlin, Heidelberg, New York: Springer.

Heider, Fritz (1958): *The Psychology of Interpersonal Relations*. New York: John Wiley & Sons.

Henle, Mary (1957 in 1986): Some Problems of Eclecticism (1957). In: M. Henle (1986), *1879 and All That. Essays in the Theory and History of Psychology*. New York: Columbia University Press, 81–92.

Henle, M. (1961): Some effects of motivational processes on cognition. In M. Henle (Ed.), *Documents   of   Gestalt Psychology* (originally in *Psychological Review, 62/6*, 1955). University of California Press, 172-186.

Henle, M. (1962): Some Aspects of the Phenomenology of the Personality. *Psychologische Beiträge*, IV(3-4), 395–404.

Henle, M. (1971/1986): The snail beneath the shell. In: *1879 and all that: Essays in the Theory and History of Psychology*, Columbia Univ Press: 1986 [orig. publ. Abraxis, Winter 1971, and in *Essays in Creativity*, North River Press: 1974]

Henle, M. (1974): On Naïve Realism. In: Robert Brodie MacLeod, Herbert L. Pick (Eds.), *Perception: Essays in Honor of James J. Gibson*. Cornell University Press, 40-56.

Henle, M. (1977/ 1986): On the Distinction Between the Phenomenal and the Physical Object, in: *1879 and all that: Essays in the Theory and History of Psychology*, Columbia Univ Press: 1986 [orig. published in in J. Nicholas, Images, Perception, and Knowledge. 1977]

Hoppe, Ferdinan (1930 in 1976): Success and Failure. (Translation of Hoppe 1930, Erfolg und Misserfolg, by Sybille Escalona). In. De Rivera 1976, 454–492.

Horvath, Adam O. & Lester Luborsky (1993): The Role of the Therapeutic Alliance in Psychotherapy. *Journal of Consulting and Clinical Psychology*, 61(4), 561–573.

Horvath, A.O. & B.D. Symonds (1991): Relation between working alliance and outcome in psychotherapy: A meta-analysis. *Journal of Counseling Psychology, 38*(2), 139–149.

Jørgensen, Carsten René (2019): *The Therapeutic Stance*. Cham/Switzerland: Springer Nature.

Jung, C. G. (1995): *Memories, dreams, reflections* (R. Winston & C. Winston, Trans.). Fontana Press.

Kahler, Taibi (1978): *Transactional Analysis Revisited*. Little Rock (Arkansas): Human Development Publications.

Karsten, Anitra (1928): Psychische Sättigung. *Psychologische Forschung*, 10, 142–154. [English translation: Karsten 1976]

Karsten, A. (1976): Mental satiation. In De Rivera 1976, 151–207.

Kästl, Rainer (2007): Gestalttheoretische Überlegungen zum psychoanalytischen Konstrukt „Übertragung". *Gestalt Theory, 29*(1), 65-73.

Kästl, R. (2011): Zur Therapeutin-Klientin-Beziehung in der Gestalttheoretischen Psychotherapie. *Phänomenal*, 3(2), 19–21.

Kästl, R. & G. Stemberger (2011): Anwendungen der Gestalttheorie in der Psychotherapie. In: H. Metz-Göckel, Hrsg., *Gestalttheoretische Inspirationen. Anwendungen der Gestalttheorie. Handbuch zur Gestalttheorie – Band 2*. Wien: Krammer, 27–70.

Katz, S.M. (2017): *Contemporary psychoanalytic field theory: stories, dreams, and metaphor*. New York: Routledge.

King, D. Brett & Michael Wertheimer (2005): *Max Wertheimer and Gestalt Theory*. New Brunswick & London: Transaction Publishers.

Koffka, Kurt (1935): *Principles of Gestalt Psychology*. New York: Harcourt-Brace.

Kohl, Kurt (1956): *Zum Problem der Sensumotorik*. Frankfurt: Waldemar Kramer.

Köhler, Wolfgang (1922): Gestaltprobleme und Anfänge einer Gestalttheorie. *Jahresbericht über d. Gesamte Physiologie 3*, 512 -39.

Köhler, W. (1929 in 1971): An Old Pseudoproblem. (Translation of W. Köhler's "Ein altes Scheinproblem" 1929, *Die Naturwissenschaften, 17*(22), 395–401, by Erich Goldmeyer). In: M. Henle (ed.), *Selected Papers of Wolfgang Köhler*, New York: Liveright, 1971, 125-141.

Köhler, W. (1938/1966): *The Place of Value in a World of Facts*. New York: Liveright. New edition 1966.

Köhler, W. (1947): *Gestalt psychology* (rev.ed.). New York: Liveright.

Köhler, W. (1957/1993): Letter to Abraham S. Luchins on the Prägnanz principle, *Gestalt Theory, 15*(3/4), 297–298.

Köhler, W. (1968): *Werte und Tatsachen*. Heidelberg: Springer. (Original 1938: *The Place of Value in a World of Facts*. New York, NY: Liveright).

Köhler, W. (1971): *Die Aufgabe der Psychologie*. Berlin-New York: De Gruyter. (Original 1969: *The Task of Gestalt Psychology*. Princeton University Press).

Kriz, Jürgen (2014): *Grundkonzepte der Psychotherapie*. 7., überarbeitete und erweiterte Auflage. Weinheim: Beltz/PVU.

Lambert, M. J. (2013; Ed.): *Bergin & Garfield's handbook of psychotherapy and behavior change* (6th Edn.). Hoboken, NJ: Wiley.

Leuner, Hanscarl (1997): *Die experimentelle Psychose. Ihre Psychopharmakologie, Phänomenologie und Dynamik in Beziehung zur Person*. Berlin: VWB.

Leuzinger-Bohleber, M. (2018): La ricchezza della ricerca psicoanalitica contemporanea: Osservazioni epistemologiche e metodologiche, alcuni esempi e il metodo di osservazione clinica a tre livelli (3LM). *Rivista di Psicoanalisi, LXIV*(2), 269-296.

Levy, E. (1943): Some Aspects of the Schizophrenic Formal Disturbance of Thought. *Psychiatry, 6*(1), 55-69.

Levy, E. (1986). A Gestalt theory of paranoia. Introduction, comment and translation of 'Heinrich Schulte'. *Gestalt Theory, 8*(4), 230-255 (Comment: 248-255).

Lewin, Kurt & Kanae Sakuma (1925): Die Sehrichtung monokularer und binokularer Objekte bei Bewegung und das Zustandekommen des Tiefeneffektes. *Psychologische Forschung, 6*, 298–357.

Lewin, K. (1926a): Vorbemerkungen über die psychischen Kräfte und die Struktur der Seele. *Psychologische Forschung, 7*(4), 294–329.

Lewin, K. (1926b): Vorsatz, Wille und Bedürfnis. *Psychologische Forschung, 7*(4), 330–385.

Lewin, K. (1928): Die Entwicklung der experimentellen Willenspsychologie und die Psychotherapie. *Archiv für Psychiatrie, 85*, 515–537.

Lewin, K. (1931): *Die psychologische Situation bei Lohn und Strafe*. Leipzig: Hirzel. Engl: The psychological situation of reward and punishment. In Lewin 1935, 114–170.

Lewin, K. (1935): *A Dynamic Theory of Personality. Selected Papers*. New York & London: McGraw-Hill.

Lewin, K. (1936): *Principles of Topological Psychology*. New York & London: McGraw-Hill.

Lewin, K., Lippitt, R. & White, R. (1939): Patterns of aggressive behaviour in experimentally created "social climates". *Journal of Social Psychology* 10, 271–299.

Lewin, K., Lippitt, R., & S.K. Escalona (1940): *Studies in topological and vector psychology* I (G. D. Stoddard, Ed.) University of Iowa studies in child welfare: Vol. 16. University of Iowa Press.

Lewin, K. (1942): Time perspective and morale. In G. Watson (Ed.), *Civilian morale*. Boston, MA: Houghton Mifflin, 48–70.

Lewin, K. (1946/1963): Behavior and development as a function of the total situation. In K. Lewin (1963), Feldtheorie in den Sozialwissenschaften. Bern: Huber, 271–329.

Lewin, K. (1951): *Field Theory in Social Science. Selected Theoretical Papers. Edited by Dorwin Cartwright*. New York: Harper & Brothers.

Lewin, K. (1951a): Field theory and learning. In Lewin 1951, 60-84.

Lewin, K. (1963/2012): *Feldtheorie in den Sozialwissenschaften*. Neuauflage 2012. Berlin: Huber.

Lewin, K. (1969): *Grundzüge der topologischen Psychologie*. Bern und Stuttgart: Verlag Hans Huber.

Lewin, K. (1982): Umweltkräfte in Verhalten und Entwicklung des Kindes (German translation of chapter III of Lewin 1935). In: K. Lewin, *Psychologie der Entwicklung und Erziehung* (Kurt-Lewin-Werke, Band 6), Bern/Huber & Stuttgart/Klett Cotta, 169-214.

Lindorfer, Bernadette & Gerhard Stemberger (2012): Unfinished Business. Die Experimente der Lewin-Gruppe zur Struktur und Dynamik von Persönlichkeit und psychologischer Umwelt. *Phänomenal*, 4(1–2), 63–70.

Lindorfer, B. (2012a): Zeigarniks Pionierstudie zum Behalten erledigter und unerledigter Handlungen. *Phänomenal*, 4(1–2), 71–73.

Lindorfer, B. (2012b): Ovsiankinas Pionierstudie zur Wiederaufnahme unterbrochener Handlungen. *Phänomenal*, 4(1–2), 74–76.

Lindorfer, B. (2017): Spannungssystem. Lexikon zur Gestalttheoretischen Psychotherapie. *Phänomenal*, 9(1), 55–57.

Lindorfer, B.; Luchins, A.S. & E.H. Luchins (2020): Der phänomenzentriert-variationale Ansatz in Forschung Psychotherapie. *Phänomenal*, 12(1), 41–50.

Lindorfer, B. (2021): Personality theory of Gestalt Theoretical Psychotherapy. Kurt Lewin's field theory and his theory of systems in tension revisited. *Gestalt Theory* 43(1), 29-46.

Lindorfer, B. (2022): Personality theory of Gestalt Theoretical Psychotherapy. Kurt Lewin's field theory and his theory of systems in tension revisited. Revised version of Lindorfer 2021. *Current volume*.

Lissner, Käte (1933): Die Entspannung von Bedürfnissen durch Ersatzhandlungen. *Psychologische Forschung*, 18, 218–250.

Luccio, Riccardo (1993): Gestalt Problems in Cognitive Psychology: Field Theory, Invariance and Auto-Organisation. In: Roberto V. (ed.), *Intelligent Perceptual Systems. Lecture Notes in Computer Science* (Lecture Notes in Artificial Intelligence), vol 745, 1-19.

Luccio, R. (2003): The Emergence of Prägnanz. Gaetano Kanizsa's Legacies. *Axiomathes*, 13, 365–387.

Luccio, R. (2019): Perceptual Simplicity: The True Role of Prägnanz and Occam. *Gestalt Theory*, 41(3), 263–276.

Luchins, Abraham S. & Edith H. Luchins (1959): *Rigidity of Behavior – A Variational Approach to the Effect of Einstellung*. Eugene, Oregon: University of Oregon Books.

Luchins, A.S. (1961): Some Aspects of Wertheimer's Approach to Personality. *Journal of Individual Psychology, 17*, 20–26.

Luchins, A.S. & E.H. Luchins, E. H. (1999): Isomorphism in Gestalt theory: Comparison of Wertheimer's and Köhler's Concepts. *Gestalt Theory, 21*(3), 208–234.

Lück, Helmut E. (1996): *Die Feldtheorie und Kurt Lewin*. Weinheim: Beltz PVU

Mahler, Wera (1933): Ersatzhandlungen verschiedenen Realitätsgrades. *Psychologische Forschung, 18*(1/2), 27-89.

Malle, Bertram F. (2008): Fritz Heider's Legacy. Celebrated Insights, Many of Them Misunderstood. *Social Psychology, 39*(3), 163–173.

Malle, B.F. (2011): Attribution theories: How people make sense of behavior. In Chadee, D. (Ed.), *Theories in social psychology*, Chichester: Wiley-Blackwell, 72-95.

Marrow, A. J. (1969): *Practical theorist – Life and work of Kurt Lewin*. New York, NY: Basic Books.

Metzger, Wolfgang (1941): *Psychologie. Die Entwicklung ihrer Grundannahmen seit Einführung des Experiments*. Dresden/Leipzig: Steinkopff (6th edition -> Metzger 2001).

Metzger, W. (1959): Die Entwicklung der Erkenntnisprozesse. In: *Handbuch der Psychologie, Bd. 3*, Göttingen: Hogrefe, 404–441.

Metzger, W. (1962/2022): *Schöpferische Freiheit*. 2. Auflage 1962 Frankfurt: Waldemar Kramer; 3. Auflage: *Schöpferische Freiheit. Gestalttheorie des Lebendigen*. Hrsg. von Marianne Soff und Gerhard Stemberger. Wien: Wolfgang Krammer.

Metzger, W. (1965 in 1986): Über die Notwendigkeit kybernetischer Vorstellungen in der Theorie des Verhaltens (1965). In Metzger 1986, 264–268.

Metzger, Wolfgang (1967/2018): Kritischer Realismus ist unbequem [Auszug aus: Der Geltungsbereich gestalttheoretischer Ansätze, Metzger 1986, 134ff]. *Phänomenal, 10*(1), 35-37.

Metzger, W. (1969 in 1986): Die Wahrnehmungswelt als zentrales Steuerungsorgan (1969). In Metzger 1986, 269–279.

Metzger, W. (1972): The Phenomenal-Perceptual Field as a Central Steering Mechanism. Lecture at the 2nd Banff Conference 1969. In: J.R. Royce & W.W. Rozeboom (eds.): *The Psychology of Knowing*, New York/Paris/London: Gordon and Breach 1972, 241-265. [English version of Metzger 1969 in 1986]

Metzger, W. (1975 in 1986): Gestalttheorie und Gruppendynamik (1975). In Metzger 1986, 210-226.

Metzger, W. (1975): *Gesetze des Sehens*. 3. Auflage. Frankfurt: Waldemar Kramer.

Metzger, W. (1976): *Psychologie in der Erziehung*. 3. Auflage. Bochum: Ferdinand Kamp.

Metzger, W. (1977 in 1986): Adler als Autor (1977). In Metzger 1986, 478-493.

Metzger, W. (1986): *Gestalt-Psychologie. Ausgewählte Werke aus den Jahren 1950 bis 1982, herausgegeben und eingeleitet von M. Stadler und H. Crabus*. Frankfurt: Waldemar Kramer.

Metzger, W. (2001): *Psychologie. Die Entwicklung ihrer Grundannahmen seit der Einführung des Experiments*. 6. Auflage. Wien: Krammer.

Metz-Göckel, Hellmuth (2014). Über Bezugsphänomene: Wie ein Sachverhalt durch den Bezug auf einen anderen seine besonderen Merkmale erhält. *Gestalt Theory, 36*(4), 355-386.

Metz-Göckel, H. (2016): *Gestalttheorie und kognitive Psychologie*. Wiesbaden: Springer.

Michotte, Albert (1950a): The Emotions Regarded as Functional Connections. In M. L. Reymert (ed.), *Feelings and Emotions: The Mooseheart Symposium*, New York: Mc Graw-Hill, 114-126, also in Michotte 1962a, 128-144.

Michotte, A. (1950b): La préfiguration dans les données sensorielles de notre conception spontanée du monde physique. In: *Proceedings and Papers of the XIIth Congress of Psychology*, Edinburgh: Oliver and Boyd, 20-22, also in Michotte 1962a, 541-544.

Michotte, A. (1951): La perception de la function "outil". In: *Essays in Psychology Dedicated to David Katz*, Uppsala: Almqvist and Wiksells, 193-213, also in Michotte 1962a, 145-167.

Michotte, A. (1954): *La perception de la causalité*. Louvain: Publications Universitaires.

Michotte, A. (1955a): L'influence de l'expérience sur la structuration des données sensorielles dans la perception. In: *Actes du XIIéme Symposium de l'Association de Psychologie Scientifique de Langue Francaise*, Paris: Presses Universitaires de France, 31-45, also in Michotte 1962a, 545-560.

Michotte, A. (1955b): Perception and Cognition. *Acta Psychologica, XI*, 70-91, also in Michotte 1962a, 561-587.

Michotte, A. (1959): Réflexions sur le role du language dans l'analyse des organisations perceptives. *Acta Psychologica, XV*, 17-34, also in Michotte 1962a, 588-609.

Michotte, A. (1962): *Causalité, permanence et réalité phénoménales*. Louvain: Publications Universitaires.

Michotte, A. (1963): *The Perception of Causality*. (English translation of Michotte 1954 by T. R. Miles & Elaine Miles.) New York: Basic Books.

Michotte, A. (1982): *Gesammelte Werke, Band 1: Die phänomenale Kausalität*. Herausgegeben von O. Heller & W. Lohr. Bern: Huber.

Montaigne, M. de (1942): *Essays*. Tr. by E. J. Trechmann (Vol. 1). New York, NY: Oxford University Press.

Neumann, Erich (1969/1990): *Depth psychology and a new ethic*. Boston: Shambala. [orig. published New York Putnam's 1969]

Norcross, John C. & Newman, C. F. (2003): Psychotherapy integration. Setting the context. In: Norcross, J. C. & M. R. Goldfried (Eds.), Handbook of psychotherapy integration. New York & Oxford: Oxford University Press, 3-45.

Norcross, John C. (2011): *Psychotherapy relationships that work. Evidence-based Responsiveness* (2nd ed.). Oxford: University Press.

Norcross, J.C. & Wampold Bruce E. (2011): Evidence-based therapy relationships: Research conclusions and clinical practices. In: Norcross J.C. (Ed.) *Psychotherapy Relationships That Work II*. New York: Oxford University Press, 423–430.

Norcross, J.C. & Lambert, M.J. (2018): Psychotherapy Relationships That Work III. *Psychotherapy, 55*(4), 303–315.

Nuttin, Joseph & Willy Lens (1985): *Future time perspective and motivation: Theory and research method*. Leuven, Belgium: Leuven University Press; Hillsdale, NJ: Erlbaum.

Ogden, Thomas H. (2009): *Rediscovering Psychoanalysis. Thinking and Dreaming, Learning and Forgetting.* Hove, East Sussex: Routledge.

Orlinsky, D.E. & Howard, K.J. (1986): Process and outcome in psychotherapy. In: Garfield, S.L. & Bergin, A.E. (Ed.), *Handbook of Psychotherapy and Behavior Change.* New York: Wiley, 311–384.

Ovsiankina, Maria (1928): Die Wiederaufnahme unterbrochener Handlungen. *Psychologische Forschung*, 11, 302–379. [English translation: Rickers-Ovsiankina 1976].

Perls, Frederick S., Hefferline, Ralph F. & Paul Goodman (1951): *Gestalt Therapy.* New York: The Julian Press.

Petzold, Hilarion G. (1992): *Integrative Therapie. Modelle, Theorien und Methoden für eine schulenübergreifende Psychotherapie. Band 2: Klinische Theorie.* Paderborn: Junfermann.

Petzold, H.G. (2011): Integrative Therapie. In Stumm 2011, 267-276.

Pfammatter, M., Junghan, U.M. & Tschacher, W. (2012): Allgemeine Wirkfaktoren der Psychotherapie: Konzepte, Widersprüche und eine Synthese. *Psychotherapie*, 17(1), 17–31.

Pieringer, W. & Fazekas, Ch. (1996): Die vier primären Erkenntnismethoden als wissenschaftliche Leitlinien für die Selbsterfahrung in der Psychotherapieausbildung. *Psychotherapie Forum*, 4(4), 229-238.

Ragsdale, Edward S. (2010): Review of Georges Wollants (2008): Gestalt Therapy: Therapy of the Situation. *Gestalt Theory*, 32(1), 93–98.

Ragsdale, E.S. (2021): Relational Determination in Interpersonal and Intrapsychic Experience. *Gestalt Theory*, 43(1), 121 – 141.

Ragsdale, E.S. (2022): Relational Determination in Interpersonal and Intrapsychic Experience. Revised version of Ragsdale 2021. *Current volume.*

Rainio, Kullervo (2009): Kurt Lewin's Dynamical Psychology Revisited and Revised. *Dynamical Psychology*, 1/2009, 1–20.

Rausch, Edwin (1979 in 1992): Neun Wünsche an die Zukunft der Psychologie (Nachdruck von 1979). *Gestalt Theory*, 14(2), 143-144.

Rausch, E. (1982): *Bild und Wahrnehmung. Psychologische Studien ausgehend von den Graphiken Volker Bußmanns.* Frankfurt: Waldemar Kramer.

Reich, Günter & Manfred Cierpka (2001, Hrsg.): *Psychotherapie der Essstörungen.* Stuttgart: Thieme.

Reich, G., v. Boetticher, Antje von (2017): *Hungern, um zu leben – die Paradoxie der Magersucht.* Gießen: Psychosozial-Verlag.

Rickers-Ovsiankina, Maria (1976): The resumption of interrupted activities. (Translation of Ovsiankina 1928) In: De Rivera 1976, 49–110.

Rogers, Carl R. (1959): A Theory of Therapy, Personality, and Interpersonal Relationships, as Developed in the Client-centered Framework. In S. Koch (ed.) *Psychology: A Study of a Science. Vol. 3: Formulations of the Person and the Social Context.* New York: McGraw Hill, 184–256.

Ruh, Michael (1999): Diagnosis in Gestalt Theoretical Psychotherapy: Map or Territory? *Studies in Gestalt Therapy*, 8, 292-293.

Sandell, R., Lazar, A., Grant, J., Carlsson, J., Schubert, J. & Broberg, J. (2006): Therapist attitudes and patient outcomes. III. A latent class analysis of therapists. *Psychological Psychotherapy*, 79(4), 629–647.

Scheler, Max (1923): *Wesen und Formen der Sympathie. Zweite, vermehrte und durchgesehene Auflage der „Phänomenologie der Sympathiegefühle"*. Bonn: Verlag von Friedrich Cohen.

Schulte, H. (1924 in 1986): An Attempt at a Theory of the Paranoid Ideas of Reference and Delusion Formation. (Translation of Schulte 1924 by E. Levy) *Gestalt Theory, 8*(4), 231–248.

Schulte, H. (1924/2002): Versuch einer Theorie der paranoischen Eigenbeziehung und Wahnbildung. *Psychologische Forschung, 5*, 1–23. Reprint in Stemberger 2002, 27–54. (Full English translation: Levy 1986)

Selvini Palazzoli, Mara (1984): *Magersucht. Von der Behandlung einzelner zur Familientherapie*. Stuttgart: Klett.

Sliosberg, Sarah (1934): Zur Dynamik des Ersatzes in Spiel- und Ernstsituationen. *Psychologische Forschung, 19*, 122–181.

Slunecko, Thomas (1996): Einfalt oder Vielfalt in der Psychotherapie. In: Pritz, A. (Hrsg.), *Psychotherapie – eine neue Wissenschaft vom Menschen*. Wien: Springer, 293-321.

Soff, Marianne & Michael Ruh (2006): Gestalttheorie und Individualpsychologie – eine fruchtbare Verbindung. *Gestalt Theory, 21*(4), 256–274.

Soff, M. (2013): Gestalt Theory and the Field of Educational Psychology: An Example. *Gestalt Theory, 35*(1), 47–58.

Soff, M. (2017): *Gestalttheorie für die Schule. Unterricht, Erziehung und Lehrergesundheit aus einer klassischen psychologischen Perspektive*. Wien: Krammer.

Soff, M. (2018): Gestalttheorie und Feldtheorie. In M. Hochgerner et al. (Hrsg.), *Gestalttherapie*. Zweite Auflage. Wien, Austria: Facultas, 13–43.

Spagnuolo-Lobb, Margherita (2010): The therapeutic relationship in Gestalt therapy. In Jacobs, L. & Hycner, R. (eds., 2010). *Relational Approaches in Gestalt Therapy*. Santa Cruz, CA: Gestalt Press, 111–129.

Staemmler, Frank-M. (2005): A babylonian confusion? On the uses and meanings of the term "field." *British Gestalt Journal*, 15(2), 64–83.

Steiner, Claude M. (1997): *Achieving Emotional Literacy*. New York: Avon Books.

Stemberger, Gerhard (2002, Hrsg.): *Psychische Störungen im Ich-Welt-Verhältnis. Gestalttheorie und psychotherapeutische Krankheitslehre*. Wien: Krammer.

Stemberger, G. (2008): Diagnostics in Gestalt Theoretical Psychotherapy. In: Bartuska et al. (Eds, 2008): *Psychotherapeutic Diagnostics – Guidelines for the new standard*. New York: Springer, 97–108.

Stemberger, G. (2009): Feldprozesse in der Psychotherapie. Der Mehr-Felder-Ansatz im diagnostischen und therapeutischen Prozess. *Phänomenal, 1*(1), 12–19.

Stemberger, G. (2010a): Dynamische Eigenheiten einer depressiven Symptomatik. *Gestalt Theory, 32*(4), 343–374.

Stemberger, G. (2010b): Mary Henles Beitrag zur Gestalttheorie der Person. *Phänomenal, 2*(2), 44–50.

Stemberger, G. (2011a): Gestalttheoretische Psychotherapie. In Stumm 2011, 218-227.

Stemberger, G. (2011b): Grundzüge der Gestalttheoretischen Psychotherapie. *Phänomenal, 3*(2), 12–18.

Stemberger, G. (2013): Eine Besonderheit der psychotherapeutischen Situation. *Phänomenal, 5*(1–2), 27–31.

Stemberger, G. (2014): Gestalttheoretische Aspekte der „Arbeit mit dem leeren Stuhl". *Phänomenal, 6*(1), 30-38.

Stemberger, G. (2016): Phänomenologie treiben. *Phänomenal, 8*(1), 30–35.

Stemberger, G. (2017a). Machtfelder in der Psychotherapie, Teil 2. *Phänomenal, 9*(1), 17–26.

Stemberger, G. (2017b): Arbeiten mit Machtfeldern. *Phänomenal, 9*(1), 26–29.

Stemberger, G. (2018a): Therapeutische Beziehung und therapeutische Praxis. Praxeologie der Gestalttheoretischen Psychotherapie, Teil 1. *Phänomenal, 10*(2), 20-28.

Stemberger, G. (2018b): A Gestalt Psychologist´s Views on Therapeutic Relationships. Lecture at the VIII° Colloquio di Etica, "L'umano e le sue potenzialità, tra cura e narrazione", Università di Macerata, March 14th, 2018.

Stemberger, G. (2018c): Über die Fähigkeit, an zwei Orten gleichzeitig zu sein. Ein Mehr-Felder-Ansatz zum Verständnis menschlichen Erlebens. *Gestalt Theory, 40*(2), 207–223.

Stemberger, G. & K. Sternek (2019): Gestalttheorie und Gefühl in neun Bildern. *Phänomenal, 11*(2), 21–28.

Stemberger, G. (2019a): Therapeutische Beziehung und therapeutische Praxis in der Gestalttheoretischen Psychotherapie (Teil 2). *Phänomenal, 11*(1), 29–34.

Stemberger, G. (2019b): Therapeutische Beziehung und therapeutische Praxis in der Gestalttheoretischen Psychotherapie (Teil 3). *Phänomenal, 11*(2), 42–50.

Stemberger, G. (2019c): 40 Jahre Gestalttheoretische Psychotherapie haben eine Konstante - Zum 70. Geburtstag von Rainer Kästl. *Phänomenal, 11*(1), 53–61.

Stemberger, G. (2019d): Some remarks on the field concept in Gestalt psychology. Chapter in: Trombini, G., Corazza, A. & G. Stemberger, G. (2019). Manifest Dream / Association Comparison: A Criterion to Monitor the Psychotherapeutic Field. Part 1. *Gestalt Theory, 41*(1), 61–78.

Stemberger, G. (2020a): Does a Society for Gestalt Theory and Its Applications Still Fit in Our Time? *Gestalt Theory, 42*(1), 63–70.

Stemberger, G. (2020b): Il punto di vista sulle relazioni terapeutiche di uno psicologo gestaltista. In: *L'umano e le sue potenzialità, tra cura e narrazione. A cura di Luigi Alici, Paola Nicolini,* Roma: Aracne Editrice, 29-45.

Stemberger, G. (2021): Ego and Self in Gestalt Theory. *Gestalt Theory, 43*(1), 47-67.

Stemberger, G. (2021b): Psychologische Situation. Lexikon zur Gestalttheoretischen Psychotherapie, *Phänomenal, 13*(2), 53–56.

Stemberger, G. (2022a): Ego and Self in Gestalt Theory. Revised version of Stemberger 2021. *Current volume.*

Stemberger, G. (2022b): Re-Organizing One's World. The Gestalt psychological Multiple-Field-Approach to "Mind-Wandering". In: N. Dario & L. Taddeo (eds.), *New Perspectives on Mind-wandering in Education,* Springer (in press).

Sternek, K. (2007): Attachment Theory and Gestalt Psychology. *Gestalt Theory, 29*(4), 310-318.

Sternek, K. (2014): Über den Einsatz und die Wirkungsweise von "Bildschirm-Techniken". *Phänomenal, 6*(1), 20-29.

Sternek, K. (2016): Intrusionen und Flashbacks (aus gestalttheoretischer Sicht). *Phänomenal, 8*(2), 53–55.

Sternek, K. (2018): Vom Nutzen erkenntnistheoretischer Modelle für die Psychotherapie. *Phänomenal, 10*(1), 15-24.

Sternek, K. (2020): Bezugssystem. Lexikon zur Gestalttheoretischen Psychotherapie. *Phänomenal, 12*(2), 57-59.

Sternek, K. (2021): Critical Realism: The Epistemic Position of Gestalt Theoretical Psychotherapy. *Gestalt Theory, 42*(3), 13–28.

Sternek, K. (2022): Critical Realism: The Epistemic Position of Gestalt Theoretical Psychotherapy. Revised version of Sternek 2021. *Current volume.*

Sternek, Katharina (2018): Vom Nutzen erkenntnistheoretischer Modelle für die Psychotherapie. *Phänomenal, 10*(1), 15-24.

Stolarski, M.; N. Fieulaine & W. van Beek (2015, eds.): *Time Perspective Theory; Review, Research and Application. Essays in Honor of Philip G. Zimbardo.* Cham Heidelberg New York Dordrecht London: Springer.

Strunk, Guido & Günter Schiepek (2014): *Therapeutisches Chaos.* Göttingen: Hogrefe.

Stumm, Gerhard (2011, Hrsg.): *Psychotherapie. Schulen und Methoden. Eine Orientierungshilfe für Theorie und Praxis.* 3. Auflage. Wien: Falter.

Stumm, G. (2011a): Einleitung. In Stumm 2011, 10-34.

Stumm, G. (2011b): Systemische Verfahren. In Stumm 2011, 251-252.

Taubner, Svenja; Kächele, Horst; Visbeck, Annette; Rapp, Andreas & Rolf Sandell (2010): Therapeutic attitudes and practice patterns among psychotherapy trainees in Germany. *European Journal of Psychotherapy and Counselling, 12*(4), 361–381.

Thinès, Georges; Costall, Alan & George Butterworth (1991, eds.): *Michotte's Experimental Phenomenology of Perception.* Hillsdale (New Jersey): Lawrence Erlbaum Associates.

Tholey, P. (1980/2018): Erkenntnistheoretische und systemtheoretische Grundlagen der Sensumotorik aus gestalttheoretischer Sicht. *Sportwissenschaften, 10*, 7-33. Reprint in Tholey 2018, 35–48.

Tholey, P. (1986/2018): Deshalb Phänomenologie! *Gestalt Theory* 8(2), 144–163. Reprint in Tholey 2018, 244-268.

Tholey, P. (1989): Overview of the Development of Lucid Dream Research in Germany. *Lucidity Letter, 8*(2), 1–30.

Tholey, P. (1990): Applications of Lucid Dreaming in Sports. *Lucidity Letter, 9*(2), 1–11.

Tholey, P. (1996): Zur Einführung. In Walter 1996, 11–15.

Tholey, P. (1998): Feldtheorien in Biologie, Biophysik, Psychologie und Sozialwissenschaften. Ein bisher unveröffentlichter Kommentar (1995) aus dem Nachlass von Paul Tholey. *ÖAGP-Informationen, 7*(5), iii–ix.

Tholey, P. (2018): *Gestalttheorie von Sport, Klartraum und Bewusstsein. Ausgewählte Arbeiten, herausgegeben und eingeleitet von G. Stemberger.* Wien: Krammer.

Trombini, Elena & Giancarlo Trombini (2006): Focal Play-Therapy in the extended child-parents context. A clinical case. *Gestalt Theory, 28*(4), 375–388.

Trombini, G. (2010): Monitorare la dinamica relazionale in psicoterapia: confronto tra sogno e associazioni. *Medicina Psicosomatica, 55*(4), 165-173.

Trombini, G. (2014): Transferential relationships as field phenomena. The relationship dynamics in the light of the manifest dream. *Gestalt Theory, 36*(1), 43-68.

Trombini, G. (2015): La dinamica transferale alla luce del sogno manifesto e delle associazioni. *Rivista di Psicoanalisi 61*(1), 45-64.

Trombini, G.; Corazza, A.; Stemberger, G. (2019): Manifest Dream/Association Comparison: A Criterion to Monitor the Psychotherapeutic Field. *Gestalt Theory, 41*(1), 61-77; *41*(3), 241-261.

Verstegen, I. (2012): True Realism Requires Representations: Enactivism versus Gestalt Theory. Published in Italian in Fiorenza Toccafondi, ed., *Filosofia e scienza. Punti d'incontro passati e presenti* (Firenze, Le Lettere, 2012). English version accessible online at https://www.academia.edu/2478577/

Wagner, E. (2007): Epistemologie. In: Stumm & Pritz (Hrsg.), *Wörterbuch der Psychotherapie*. Wien: Springer, 169.

Waldvogel, Bruno (1992): *Psychoanalyse und Gestaltpsychologie*. Stuttgart: Frommann-Holzboog.

Walter, H.-J. P. (1977): Gestalttheorie und Psychotherapie. Ein Beitrag zur theoretischen Begründung der integrativen Anwendung von Gestalt-Therapie, Psychodrama, Gesprächstherapie, Tiefenpsychologie, Verhaltenstherapie und Gruppendynamik. Darmstadt: Steinkopff.

Walter, H.-J. P. (1985/1994): *Gestalttheorie und Psychotherapie. Zur integrativen Anwendung zeitgenössischer Therapieformen*. Opladen: Westdeutscher Verlag.

Walter, H.-J. P. (1996): *Angewandte Gestalttheorie in Psychotherapie und Psychohygiene*. Opladen: Westdeutscher Verlag.

Walter, H.-J. P. (1997): Cognitive Behavior Therapy and Gestalt Theoretical Psychotherapy. *Gestalt! a chronicle of the developing application of Gestalt principles, 1*(1).

Walter, H.-J. P. (1999): What do Gestalt therapy and Gestalt theory have to do with each other? *The Gestalt Journal, XXII*(1), 45-68.

Walter, H.-J. P. (2001): Zur Bedeutung der Begriffe „Physikalisch", „Transphänomenal" und „Wirklichkeit im 1. Sinne". *Gestalt Theory, 23*(2), 102-112.

Wedam, Uta (2007): Relations and Structures - Psychotherapeutic Care with Traumatized Refugees. *Gestalt Theory, 29*(4). 302-309.

Weiner, I. B., Millon, T., & Lerner, M. J. (2003, eds.): *Handbook of psychology, Vol. 5, Personality and Social Psychology*. Hoboden, NJ: John Wiley & Sons.

Wertheimer, Max (1923 in 2012): Untersuchungen zur Lehre von der Gestalt. II. *Psychologische Forschung*, 4, 1923, 301–350. Full translation into English 2012 by Michael Wertheimer and Karen W. Watkins: Investigations on Gestalt Principles. In: L. Spillmann (ed.), *Max Wertheimer: On Perceived Motion and Figural Organization*, Cambridge/Mass. & London: The MIT Press, 127-182.

Wertheimer, M. (1924 in 1944): Gestalt Theory. Translation of "Über Gestalttheorie" (Address, by MW, before the Kant Society, Berlin, 17th December, 1924) by N. Nairn-Allis, *Social Research, 11*(1), 81-99. An abridged translation has been published earlier in: W.D. Ellis (1938), *Source Book of Gestalt Psychology*, New York: Harcourt, Brace and Co., 1-11.

Wertheimer, M. (1945/2020): *Productive Thinking*. New York: Harper. New edition 2020, edited by Viktor Sarris: Springer.

Whorf, Benjamin Lee (1956): *Language, Thought and Reality*. Cambridge (Massachusetts): MIT Press.

Wicklund, R. A., & Gollwitzer, P. M. (1981): Symbolic self-completion, attempted influence, and self-deprecation. *Basic and Applied Social Psychology, 2*(2), pp. 89–114.

Wicklund, R. A., & Gollwitzer, P. M. (1982): *Symbolic self-completion*. Hillsdale, N.J.: Lawrence Erlbaum.

Wieltschnig, Sigrid (2016): Traumatic Stress and its Impact on Body, Mind and Society. *Gestalt Theory, 38*(2/3), 311-320.

Willig, C. (2019): Ontological and epistemological reflexivity: A core skill for therapists. *Counselling and Psychotherapy Research, 19*(3), 186 – 194.

Wollants, Georges (2008/2012): *Gestalt Therapy. Therapy of the Situation*. Turnhout, Belgium: Faculteit voor Mens en Samenleving (2008). New edition 2012: Sage Publications.

Wright, H. F. (1937): The influence of barriers on the strength of motivation. Duke University. *Contributions to Psychological Theory, 1*, 3-143.

Wurmser, Léon (1993): `Grausame Rächerin´ und `gefügige Sklavin´ - Sadomasochismus, Scham und Ressentiment bei Eßstörungen. In G.H. Seidler (Hrsg.): *Magersucht. Öffentliches Geheimnis*. Vandenhoeck & Ruprecht: Göttingen, 28-52.

Zabransky, Dieter; Wagner-Lukesch, Eva; Stemberger, Gerhard & Angelika Böhm (2018): Grundlagen der Gestalttheoretischen Psychotherapie. In: M. Hochgerner et al. (Hrsg.), *Gestalttherapie*, 2., überarbeitete Auflage, Wien: Facultas, 132–169.

Zeigarnik, Bluma (1927): Über das Behalten von erledigten und unerledigten Handlungen. *Psychologische Forschung, 9*, 1–85.

Zimbardo, P. G., & Boyd, J. N. (1999): Putting time in perspective: A valid, reliable individual-differences metric. *Journal of Personality and Social Psychology, 77*(6), 1271–1288. Also in Stolarski et al. 2015, 17–56.

Żuczkowski, Andrzej (1995): *Strutture dell'esperienza e strutture del linguaggio*. Bologna: CLUEB.

Żuczkowski, A. (1998): Linguaggio e causalità affettiva. In: M. W. Battacchi, M. Bosinelli, P. E. Ricci Bitti, G. Trombini (eds), *Le ragioni della psicologia. Saggi in onore di Renzo Canestrari*, Milano: Franco Angeli, 113-124.

Żuczkowski, A. (1999a): Speech acts and emotional causality in everyday life. *Analecta Husserliana, LIX*, 521-532.

Żuczkowski, A. (1999b): Percezione della causalità e linguaggio. In A. Zuczkowski (ed.), *Percezione della causalità e linguaggio*, Bologna: CLUEB, 27-42.

Żuczkowski, A. (2003): I fondamenti visivi del linguaggio. In: U. Savardi and A. Mazzocco (eds.), *Figura e sfondo*, 225-238.

Żuczkowski, A. (2004): "Tu mi fai arrabbiare": linguaggio e causalità affettiva. *Rivista Italiana di Analisi Transazionale, XXIV, 10*(47), 75-84.

Żuczkowski, A. (2005): Percezione visiva e linguaggio. *Teorie e Modelli, 9*, 2-3, 107-126.

Żuczkowski, A. (2006): Koffka dialoga con Musil. *Ricerche di Psicologia, XXIX*, 3,19-38.

Żuczkowski, A. (2008): "You make me feel…": affective causality in language communication. *Proceedings of the AISB 2008 Symposium on Affective Language in Human and Machine*, University of Aberdeen, 33-36.

Żuczkowski, A. & Ilaria Riccioni (2010): Sprache und Kommunikation: Kritischer Realismus, Strukturanalyse und dialogischer Zugang. In G. Galli (Hrsg.), *Gestaltpsychologie und Person. Entwicklungen der Gestaltpsychologie*, Wien: Verlag Krammer, 109-126.

Żuczkowski, A., Bongelli, Ramona & Ilaria Riccioni (2017): *Epistemic Stance in Dialogue. Knowing, Unknowing, Believing*. Amsterdam / Philadelphia: John Benjamins Publishing Company.

Żuczkowski, A. & G. Stemberger (2022): "The way you make me feel" – Feeling-causality in language communication. *Current volume.*

About the Authors

Beneder, Doris, Mag.ª rer.nat., born in 1962. Clinical & Health Psychologist, psychotherapist and clinical supervisor; member of the teaching faculty of the Austrian Association for Gestalt Theoretical Psychotherapy (ÖAGP). Member of the psychotherapy advisory council of the Austrian Federal Ministry for Health. Co-editor of *Psychotherapie Forum* – the journal of the Austrian Federal Association for Psychotherapy (ÖBVP). Her work focuses on psychotherapeutic diagnostics and group psychotherapy. Address: ÖAGP, Fünfhausgasse 5/20, 1150 Wien, Austria. E-Mail: doris.beneder@oeagp.at

Böhm, Angelika, PhD, works as a psychotherapist and clinical supervisor as well as a member of the teaching faculty of the Austrian Association of Gestalt Theoretical Psychotherapy (ÖAGP). She holds degrees in Psychotherapy Science and in Education and is a member of the Board of Directors of the GTA (International multidisciplinary *Society of Gestalt Theory and its Applications*). Furthermore, she is co-editor of the journal for Gestalt Theoretical Psychotherapy "Phänomenal – Zeitschrift für Gestalttheoretische Psychotherapie". Address: ÖAGP, Fünfhausgasse 5/20, 1150 Wien (Vienna), Austria. Email: angelika.boehm@oeagp.at

Thomas Fuchs, PhD, is a clinical psychologist and psychotherapist working in private practice in Bonn, Germany. He is educated and trained in Psychodynamic Therapy and Gestalt Theoretical Psychotherapy, in whose further development he has played a significant role since many years. While working at the psychological department of the university in Bonn he developed and published a therapy outcome/process questionnaire (*Bonner Fragebogen für Therapie und Beratung*). His psychotherapy focus is on eating disorders, which is as well his main current research interest. His publications are foremost on the topic of eating disorders, comparing Gestalt Theoretical Psychotherapy / psychoanalysis and psychotherapy research, and on the working alliance in psychotherapy and clinical supervision. He is a longstanding member of the Board of Directors of the international multidisciplinary „Society for Gestalt Theory and its Applications" (GTA). He is associated to the teaching faculty of the Austrian Association of Gestalt Theoretical Psychotherapy (ÖAGP) and associate editor of the psychotherapy journal „Phänomenal – Zeitschrift für Gestalttheoretische Psychotherapie". Contact: thomasfuchspsycho@t-online.de

Lindorfer, Bernadette, Mag.ª phil, born in 1965. Clinical & Health Psychologist, psychotherapist and clinical supervisor; member of the teaching faculty of the Austrian Association for Gestalt Theoretical Psychotherapy (ÖAGP). Member of the ethics-committee of the psychotherapy advisory council of the Austrian Federal Ministry for Health. Co-editor of „Phänomenal – Zeitschrift für Gestalttheoretische Psychotherapie". Address: ÖAGP, Fünfhausgasse 5/20, 1150 Wien (Vienna), Austria. Email: bernadette.lindorfer@oeagp.at

Ragsdale, Edward, Ph.D., born in 1948, is a psychotherapist in New York City. He studied Gestalt theory under Mary Henle at the New School for Social Research. He has published articles exploring Gestalt theory's relation to both depth psychology and Mahayana Buddhism. He is at work on a book exploring moral polarization as an organizing principle of psyches and societies, whose further development may require reconciliation of those dualistically opposing part-contexts into a more integrated and self-aware whole. Address: 51 Fifth Avenue, #16D, New York, NY 10003, USA. Email: edragsdale@gmail.com

Stemberger, Gerhard, born 1947, Dr.phil., lives in Vienna and Berlin. He is a psychotherapist and clinical supervisor as well as a member of the teaching faculty for Gestalt Theoretical Psychotherapy of the ÖAGP. His work focuses on the history and theory of the clinical application of Gestalt theory, in particular the theoretical foundation of Gestalt Theoretical Psychotherapy. He is the former president of the Society for Gestalt Theory and its Applications (GTA), long-time editor of the journal *Gestalt Theory* and co-publisher of *Phänomenal – Zeitschrift für Gestalttheoretische Psychotherapie* (Journal for Gestalt Theoretical Psychotherapy). He is also the editor and co-author of the books *Psychische Störungen im Ich-Welt-Verhältnis* (Mental Disorders in the I-World Relationship; 2002), *Giuseppe Galli: Der Mensch als Mit-Mensch* (Man as fellow-human; 2017) and *Paul Tholey: Gestalttheorie von Sport, Klartraum und Bewusstsein* (Gestalt theory of Sports, Lucid Dreaming and Consciousness; 2018). Address: Wintergasse 75-77/7, 3002 Purkersdorf, Austria. Email: gst@gestalttheory.net

Sternek, Katharina, born in 1962, is a Gestalt-theoretical psychotherapist and clinical supervisor in Vienna. She is a member of the teaching faculty of the ÖAGP (Austrian Association of Gestalt Theoretical Psychotherapy) and a member of the advisory board of GTA (International Society of Gestalt Theory and its Applications). Furthermore, she is a member of the ethics-committee of the psychotherapy advisory council of the Austrian Federal Ministry for Health. She is co-editor of „Phänomenal – Zeitschrift für Gestalttheoretische Psychotherapie". Publications in the field of epistemology in psychotherapy, trauma therapy and related clinical topics. Address: ÖAGP, Fünfhausgasse 5/20. 1150 Wien (Vienna), Austria. Email: sternek@sternek-psychotherapie.at

Trombini, Elena, born 1962, is a Full Professor of Dynamic Psychology at the Department of Psychology of the University of Bologna, where she directs the Psychological Consultation Service for children and parents and the Research Lab for the study of Developmental Psychopathology and

Psychotherapy. She teaches Clinical Psychology and Developmental Psychopathology in the undergraduate programs of Medicine and Psychology and Education, and in postgraduate programs as well. She is a psychotherapist and a member of the Italian Psychological Association for the division of clinical and dynamic psychology. Her clinical and research activities revolve around clinical child (prematurity, eating and evacuative behavioral disorders), and adult (obesity, psychological distress and emotional intelligence, parenting) psychology with a main focus on the development of psychodiagnostic methods and psychotherapeutic intervention. She is the author of several papers published on international peer-reviewed journals and has a number of national and international research collaborations. Address: Department of Psychology "Renzo Canestrari", Viale Berti Pichat, 5, 40127 Bologna, Italy. Email: elena.trombini@unibo.it

Trombini, Giancarlo, born 1934, is an Emeritus Professor of Clinical Psychology and a Director of the Interdisciplinary Center for the Study of Psychosomatic Disorders at the University of Bologna. He is also a member of the International Psychoanalytic Association. In 1975, he was the Chair of General Psychology at the University of Padova, and in 1977, he was the first Italian Chair of Psychosomatic Medicine at the University of Bologna. He has been working for more than 30 years on psychosomatic disorders in adults and children, and he designed new psychotherapeutic methods for children (Focal Play-Therapy and Drawn Stories). Address: Department of Psychology "Renzo Canestrari", Viale Berti Pichat, 5, 40127 Bologna, Italy. Email: prof.giancarlo.trombini@gmail.com

Zuczkowski, Andrzej, born 1946, is full professor in General Psychology at the University of Macerata (Italy), Department of Education, Cultural Heritage and Tourism, where he teaches Cognitive Psychology. He is Director of the Research Centre for Psychology of Communication. He was formed in Gestalt psychology and experimental phenomenology, in linguistics and in Transactional Analysis psychotherapy. His main scientific and research interests concern the semantic interpretation of texts, the pragmatics of dialogues (professional and non-professional), the relationship between language and phenomenal reality. With regard to the third topic, he has been studying the epistemic and evidential aspects in written and spoken corpora. Address: Department of Education, Cultural Heritage and Tourism, University of Macerata, p.le L. Bertelli 1, 62100 Macerata, Italy. Email: zuko@unimc.it

Österreichische Arbeitsgemeinschaft für Gestalttheoretische Psychotherapie (ÖAGP / Austrian Association for Gestalt Theoretical Psychotherapy AAGTP): The ÖAGP/AAGTP was founded in 1985, thereby replacing a predecessor organization that had been in existence since 1979. It is a state accredited facility for specialized psychotherapy training in the method of Gestalt Theoretical Psychotherapy (GTP) in Austria. Gestalt Theoretical Psychotherapy is officially recognized in Austria as a scientifically based psychotherapy method in its own right besides others like psychoanalysis, individual psychology, analytical psychology, behavior therapy, psychodrama, logotherapy and existential analysis, Integrative Gestalt therapy, Integrative Therapy, Rogerian person-centered psychotherapy, systemic family therapy and others. In addition, the ÖAGP/AAGTP is the professional association of psychotherapists practicing this method in Austria and promotes the application and further development of Gestalt theory in the field of psychotherapy. The international scientific umbrella organization of ÖAGP/AAGTP is the multidisciplinary *Society for Gestalt Theory and its Applications* (GTA). The scientific journal of the GTA is the international multidisciplinary journal *Gestalt Theory*. In addition, ÖAGP has been publishing the journal *Phänomenal - Zeitschrift für Gestalttheoretische Psychotherapie* (Verlag Krammer, Vienna), a journal specialized in psychotherapy, since 2009.